Early Intervention Studies for Young Children with Special Needs

Edited by DAVID MITCHELL AND ROY I. BROWN

Both at Department of Rehabilitation Studies, University of Calgary, Canada

Chapman and Hall
London . New York . Tokyo . Melbourne . Madras

UK   Chapman and Hall, 2–6 Boundary Row, London SE1 8HN
USA   Chapman and Hall, 29 West 35th Street, New York NY10001
Japan   Chapman and Hall Japan, Thomson Publishing Japan,
            Hirakawacho Nemoto Building, 7F, 1-7-11 Hirakawa-cho,
            Chiyoda-ku, Tokyo 102
Australia   Chapman and Hall Australia, Thomas Nelson Australia,
            102 Dodds Street, South Melbourne, Victoria 3205
India   Chapman and Hall India, R. Seshadri, 32 Second Main Road,
            CIT East, Madras 600 035

First edition 1991

© 1991 David Mitchell and Roy I. Brown

Printed in Great Britain by Page Bros (Norwich) Ltd

ISBN 0–412–31530–0

British Library Cataloguing in Publication Data
Early intervention studies for young children with special
    needs. — (Rehabilitation education).
    1. Handicapped children. Development
    I. Mitchell, David *1940–*   II. Brown, Roy I. (Roy Irwin)
    1933–   III. Series
    155.45
    ISBN 0–412–31530–0

Library of Congress Cataloguing-in-Publication Data
Available

CONTENTS

Roy Brown, Professor of Educational Psychology and Director, Rehabilitation Studies Programme, University of Calgary, Calgary, Canada

Ron Neufeld, Director, Field Development Office, Faculty of Education, University of British Columbia, Vancouver, Canada

Len Barton, Head of Academic and Professional Development, Bristol Polytechnic, Bristol, United Kingdom

Robert Heath, Research Psychologist, Centre for the Development of Early Education, Hawaii, U.S.A.

Paula Levin, Lecturer in Educational Research, Teacher Education Program, University of California, San Diego, U.S.A.

Contents

LIST OF CONTRIBUTORS

Dr. R. L. Brown
Rehabilitation Studies Programme
University of Calgary
2500 University Drive N.W.
Calgary, Alberta
T2N 1N4 Canada

Dr. D. M. Mitchell
Education Department
University of Waikato
Private Bag
Hamilton
New Zealand

Dr. G. R. Neufeld
Faculty of Education
Distance Education Office
University of British Columbia
2125 Main Mall
Vancouver, British Columbia
V6T 1Z5 Canada

Dr. K. Barton
Bristol Polytechnic
Redland Hill
Bristol, BS6 6UZ
United Kingdom

Drs. R. Heath and P. Levine
Research Psychologists
Center for the Development of Early Eduation
Kamehameha Schools
Bernice Pauahi Bishop Estate
1850 Makuakane Street
Honolulu, Hawaii 98617
United States

Dr. R. Ferguson
School of Child and Youth Care
University of Victoria
Victoria, British Columbia
V8W 2Y2
Canada

Dr. R. Serpell
Department of Psychology
Baltimore County Campus
University of Maryland
5401 Wilkens Avenue
Baltimore, Maryland 21228
United States

Dr. K. D. Ballard
University of Otago
P.O. Box 56
Dunedin
New Zealand

Drs. A. Nortari, K. Slentz and D. Bricker
Center on Human Development
Division of Special Education and
Rehabilitation
Clinical Services Building
College of Education
Eugene, Oregon 97403-1211
United States

Dr. G. Hornby
Education Department
University of Hull
Cottingham Road
Hull, HU6 7RX
United Kingdom

Drs. P. Price and S. Bochner
Special Education Centre
Macquarie University
North Ryde, New South Wales 2109
Australia

Drs. R. Simeonsson and D. Bailey
Frank Porter Graham Child Development
Center
University of North Carolina at Chapel Hill
CB No. 8180
Highway 54 Bypass West
Chapel Hill, North Carolina 27599-8180
United States

ACKNOWLEDGEMENTS

The suggestion for this jointly edited book came from David Mitchell. Design and development have been joint responsibilities of the editors. In attempting to ensure a reasonably integrated approach each chapter has received a detailed edit from one of us with a second edit with suggested changes from the other editor. The chapter authors have responded to these suggestions and we would like to thank them for their courteous and detailed responses. We believe this has raised the quality of the book. Nevertheless, we recognize there are some overlapping ideas and we have left these alone believing they are necessary for the logical development of a chapter or they demonstrate common themes that are developing within the field of early intervention.

We wish to acknowledge the major assistance of Kathryn Nikolaychuk who typed the manuscript on word processor and did much to identify inappropriate wording or inconsistent editing — a challenge when authors come from diverse backgrounds. We also wish to thank Aimée Anderson, Linda Culshaw and Pat Udberg who also contributed to the initial word processing task. John Kordyback was responsible for setting the figures on computer. We also wish to thank him for solving some of the challenges of printing the master copy. Finally, we acknowledge the patience and support of Ms Christine Birdsall and Ms Terri Cooper of Routledge, Chapman and Hall, and not least for their understanding patience in awaiting our final text.

D.R.M.
R.I.B.
1989

PREFACE

This is the fourth volume in the Rehabilitation Education Series. It is the first volume to be co-edited and follows a volume on quality of life. The first few years of a child's life sets the pattern for many issues associated with quality of life. Although intervention may at later stages enhance quality of life, it is in these first years that the attitudes and systems of society can have long lasting effects. The early years are increasingly seen as the province of the educator and in children with disabilities, special education. They are already recognized as the province of the health professional. Here we attempt to take a different line re-inforcing the idea that child and family are the interacting system we serve. The needs are often multidisciplinary, but we need to recognize context as the critical marker. Thus assessment needs to be linked to program-mes and therefore programmes themselves have to be evaluated, and environmental issues underlined. In particular the contribu-tion from those with sociological interests are noted. Intervention, whether it be psychological or educational, is frequently and ideally placed in the hands of parents or the nearest caregiver. The professional becomes the processor ever mindful of the context in which needs and goals are experienced. These issues are basic to the issues of quality of life.

D.R.M.
R.I.B.
1989

INTRODUCTION AND OVERVIEW

During the past decade or so, many countries have seen a rapid expansion of early intervention provisions for infants and toddlers with special needs. These developments reflect a confluence of several factors. Firstly, there has been a growing awareness of the importance of early experiences for the development of individuals, especially those who have special needs which arise from disabilities or risk factors. Secondly, the shift away from institutionalization towards community care, which is proceeding apace in many societies, is leading parents to seek regular professional assistance in caring for and educating their children with disabilities before they enter the school system. Thirdly, there is a growing recognition that infants and toddlers with special needs have a right to equal opportunities to develop their potential. The result of these trends has been that in some countries early intervention programmes are gaining increasing acceptance as part of the range of human services to which families should have access. Nowhere is this better reflected than in the United States where recent legislation (PL 99-457) has mandated statewide, comprehensive interagency programmes of early intervention services for infants and toddlers with handicaps and their families.

The rapid expansion of early intervention programmes does not necessarily reflect a consensus among service providers as to what comprises an optimal service model. Indeed, existing programmes are quite diverse with respect to their policies and practices in a whole range of areas, even in countries operating under quite explicit legislative guidelines. Thus, there is heterogeneity in terms of the agencies which control programmes, their clientele, their mode of service delivery, assessment methods, curriculum design, cultural sensitivity, staff training, relationships with parents, evaluation procedures, approaches to advocacy, and so on. Despite these variations in practice, there is a growing consensus among researchers and practitioners alike as to what constitutes sound criteria for planning high quality early intervention programmes. This book represents an attempt to crystallize these criteria and provides examples of good practice drawn from research and from programmes in several countries.

For the purposes of this book, early intervention is defined as systematic strategies aimed at promoting the optimal development of infants and toddlers with special needs and at enhancing the functioning of their families or caregivers. Expressed another way, the overall aim of early intervention is to employ preventive strategies to reduce the occurrence and/or the severity of disabling or handicapping conditions in infants and toddlers. Preventive strategies can be considered at two different levels: primary and secondary. Primary prevention is concerned with averting the conditions which give rise to disabilities or handicaps. This involves consideration of such factors as immunization (e.g. against poliomyelitis), genetic counselling (e.g. to reduce the risk of some types of Down's Syndrome), public health measures (e.g. campaigns to discourage smoking or alcohol consumption during pregnancy), social engineering (e.g. to reduce poverty), or educational measures (e.g. to help adolescents acquire parenting skills). Chapters which include consideration of primary prevention strategies include Chapter 1 in which the risks arising from such factors as nutritional inadequacies, marriage amongst family members and poor standards of public health in developing countries are outlined, Chapters 3 and 4 where there is a discussion of the significance of cultural and social factors on disability and its identification, and Chapter 5 which deals with such issues as malnutrition and social interaction patterns between mothers and infants in Third World countries. The main focus of this book, however, is on secondary prevention. This has to do with the early identification of conditions which are likely to place a child's development at serious risk, and the institution of measures to ameliorate or reduce the severity of any disability or handicap which might result from such factors. Within this broad context most of the chapters consider such themes as normalization (Chapters 1, 2, and 12), the empowerment of parents or advocates (Chapters 1, 2, 3, 4, 5, 8, 11 and 12), the assessment of children and their families (Chapters 1, 5, 6, 7, 11 and 12), the design of curriculum (Chapters 7, 9 and 12), family involvement in early intervention (Chapters 2, 3, 4, 5, 6, 8, 9, 10, 11, and 12), the importance of cultural sensitivity (Chapters 4 and 12), the significance of community attitudes towards disability (Chapters 1, 2, and 3), the training of professionals to work in the field of intervention (Chapters 4, 5, 8, 10 and 12), and the evaluation of early intervention programmes (Chapters 4, 11 and 12). Special needs covers factors which range from manifest disabilities to 'risk' features arising from biological and/or environmental factors. Broadly, these needs arise from difficulties that some infants and toddlers have in processing the various aspects of their environments. For some, the difficulties are in dealing with the linguistic challenges, for others there may be problems in physically negotiating or inadequately sensing their environments, while for still others their difficulties may be in accessing the mainstream culture of their communities. Many face complex challenges which represent an interaction of these difficulties. In degree, the problems vary from the profoundest degree of severity to those that are relatively mild, but are nevertheless of concern to family members. It should therefore be recognized that the term special needs covers a very wide range of behaviours and characteristics. In this book, although writers will illustrate some of their points with reference to particular categories of disability, for the most party they adopt a non-categorical approach. This is not to say that there is no utility in attempting to adapt programmes to take account of particular categories of special needs among infants and toddlers, but rather to emphasize the commonality of approaches to working with such children.

This book is intended to provide a reference for students, professionals, parents and administrators who are, or will be, directly involved in establishing, operating or evaluating early intervention programmes for infants and toddlers with special needs. The book should be particularly relevant to those in child care, rehabilitation education, social welfare and allied areas. The contributors to the book represent a blend of practical and research experience and have all fulfilled their brief to balance theoretical and research perspectives with practical examples.

As far as possible, the content of the following twelve chapters reflects a concern for advancing ideas that could be taken up in early intervention programmes around the world. To this end, the authors have been deliberately selected to provide a spread of international experience and have been drawn from several countries— Australia, Canada, New Zealand, the United Kingdom, the United States, and Zambia.

A discussion of changing concepts of disability taking a cross-cultural view of the issues involved is presented in Chapter 1. It stresses that the nomenclature in the field of disability is constantly changing and the appropriateness of fit is affected by the standards of service knowledge and research in any particular country. It is suggested that the borderline between disability and normality is artificial and that the concepts relating to underfunctioning, and consequently the need for intervention, should be expanded. This, it is suggested, is essential if the value system in a quality of life model is to be realized.

Chapter 2 is directed to parents and professionals who wish to improve the quality of service for young children with special needs by using advocacy strategies. In this chapter, advocacy is defined, a framework of beliefs and values is proposed, and a variety of advocacy approaches and activities are described.

The next chapter presents arguments suggesting that those involved in early intervention programmes should take a self-critical perspective, particularly with regard to the consideration given to the parents' viewpoint in such matters as rights, confidentiality, privacy, decision-making and social justice.

The following two chapters deal with cultural aspects of early intervention. The first of these chapters argues that a consideration of culture is critical for appropriately designing and evaluating early intervention programmes. Ways of achieving cultural pluralism — or, at the very least, cultural sensitivity — are described as impinging on all aspects of the work undertaken in early intervention programmes.

The second of these chapters is concerned with early intervention in Third World countries. This chapter takes up a range of issues including the politics of disability, the logistical difficulties of providing programmes in countries with limited educational and social service infrastructures, the importance of developing ecologically valid assessment instruments, ways of diffusing technical advice to families living in scattered rural areas, and the training of professional personnel.

In Chapter 6 an ecological perspective on assessment is examined — the strategies used to evaluate the cultural, social and physical context within which learning and development take place. The case is made for assessing young children as they interact with other persons, especially members of their families in the environments in which they learn. But most practitioners also recognize the importance of linking assessment to content and practice. This issue is taken up in Chapter 7 where the approach is to view curricula within the broader context of a programme's assessment procedures. In this chapter, assessment instruments and curricula packages that permit a linked approach are reviewed. In the next chapter the concern is with various aspects of parent involvement in early intervention programmes. In particular, there is a discussion of how parents adapt to disability, models of family functioning, examples of parent-professional partnership, and the skills needed by professionals in order to work effectively with parents. Parents' roles in working with young children with special needs are also addressed in the subsequent chapter, which focuses on the need for early intervention programmes to be concerned with facilitating mother–child interaction. This chapter includes detailed descriptions of language programmes that direct attention to strategies for assisting primary caregivers to mediate their young children's learning though ongoing interaction with them. Issues to do with the education and training of early interventional programme personnel are discussed in Chapter 10. Some of the key aspects of the practitioner role and their relationship to preservice and inservice preparation programmes are examined.

The broad issues of designing and evaluating early intervention programmes follow naturally from this and are addressed in the following two chapters. The first chapter recognizes that traditional research procedures may not be fully applicable to evaluating the impact of early intervention programmes. Rather, it is argued that an evaluation model based on the legal notion of preponderant evidence might be a more appropriate one to follow in an area which is inherently varied in precision and certainty. The second outlines several principles which should underlie programme evaluation and describes the rationale, structure and administration of an internationally validated scale for evaluating early intervention programmes.

Although these twelve chapters traverse a wide range of topics, various philosophical and theoretical themes recur. An over-riding theme — which is almost the *sine qua non* of the book — is the assumption that infants and toddlers with special needs have a right to services that will help them to develop their potential and that this is critical to any suitable expression of quality of life. Secondly, almost all of our authors have taken a social systems or ecological perspective, arguing that early intervention programmes should not be restricted to what goes on between a professional and a child with special needs, but should involve families, communities and the broader society. A third theme — and one that is not surprising in an international volume — is the case presented by many of our authors that programmes should be sensitive and responsive to cultural diversity, not only between countries, but also within countries. The final theme which unites the various chapters is the explicit or implicit recognition that early intervention is emerging as a distinct field of professional expertise. It is fundamental to any development of rehabilitation education as a generic professional area. Although it shares much with allied fields, particularly special education and rehabilitation, there are unique demands in working with infants and toddlers with special needs and their families and in establishing close collaborative relationships amongst a range of disciplines. Recognition of these requirements is increasingly leading to an acceptance that standards for professional practice must be established, that personnel should be appropriately trained for their roles and that they should be held accountable for their performance. This accountability is also an essential feature of any quality of life model and a requirement for any valued professional service.

This book then, provides a comprehensive discussion of some of the most critical issues in designing and implementing early intervention programmes for infants and toddlers with special needs and their families. Its international perspective and its concern for establishing a firm theoretical base for professional practice help to provide a framework against which existing programmes can be critically evaluated and new programmes can be developed.

D.R.M.
R.I.B.

CHANGING CONCEPTS OF DISABILITY IN
     DEVELOPED AND DEVELOPING COMMUNITIES

Roy I. Brown

INTRODUCTION

It is commonly recognized that disability results from physical,
environmental or biological factors which prevent an individual
from functioning effectively without specialized intervention or
modification of the environment. The World Programme of
Action regards handicap as a function of the relationships between
disabled persons and their environment. Handicap occurs when
an individual encounters cultural, physical or social barriers preventing his or her access to systems available to other citizens
(United Nations, 1986). Thus modifications to an environment of
a physical or social nature may reduce the handicap but not the
disability. For example, removing curbstones may make it easier
for a physically impaired person to cross the road, or a prosthetic
device which provides access to a computer terminal may improve
the range of communication or problem solving for an individual
(Ryba, 1989). Both reduce the person's handicap, without removing the disability. Although such discriminations have served as
working definitions in international circles for some time, they are
not entirely felicitous expressions of disability and handicap.
     It is recognized that many developmentally disabled per-
sons, particularly those with mental handicaps from deprived
environments, may show compensatory growth and development in their late teens and twenties which renders them less
handicapped and less disabled. The data from Clarke and Clarke
(1976) on cognitive changes in persons with mental handicaps
demonstrates this. However, it has never been completely resolved why such delays of growth occur. They may be due to
biological mechanisms which, when there is deprivation in early

1

childhood, delay the biological clock. This is implied by Bloom (1965) in relation to individuals who are nutritionally deprived but show compensatory physical growth later in life. On the other hand, compensation in the cognitive sphere may have to await the receipt of a range of environmental stimuli which ensures that basic cognitive structures can be developed. Recent studies on the relationship between psychological stimulation and brain structure suggest such an interaction is indeed possible (Brown and Hughson, 1987). Dobbing (1975) also underlines the view that plasticity and growth in brain structure is much greater and covers a greater time span than previously recognized. That major change can occur with young preschool children is shown in the work of Heber and Garber (1971). Enriched and structured environments can reduce mental handicap (Bronfenbrenner,1979), but it may be questioned whether any disability still exists.

In developing countries the situation is more confusing. There a large number of young children may be placed at risk through a variety of adverse variables such as nutritional inadequacy (Wynn and Wynn, 1981), and become susceptible to a wide range of diseases. Inadequate parenting models within the context of large families, along with social and economic hardship, can increase the incidence of prematurity and restrict early development (Birch and Gussow, 1970). The studies collated by Wynn and Wynn underline the effects of inadequate nutrition on fecundity, prematurity of birth and likelihood of brain injury. The effects may be quite subtle and cross economic strata. For example, Wynn and Wynn note that the degree of availability of fresh fruit is associated with the level of reproductive casualties. This is believed to be associated with availability of substances such as vitamin C. Its absence is associated with, for example, a high incidence of congenital malformations. The authors raise the question of how far family poverty is responsible for very low vitamin C intake by women and the extent to which low intake is a result of attitudes and poor education.

INTERPRETATION AND INTERACTION IN DISABILITY

The adverse conditions surrounding conception, birth and early development place children in developing countries at particular risk. Given that deficiencies in a very large proportion of young children can occur in a particular country, it has been questioned whether it is appropriate to regard such children as disabled, largely because in developed countries disability is defined in terms of exceptionality. It has been suggested that only those conditions which are strictly disabling through biological defect, or presumably extreme physical trauma, should be recognized as the subject of discussion. Under these circumstances the definition of disability would be limited. Prevalence would differ in form and magnitude from one country to another depending on each country's social and economic viability and the inhabitants' susceptibility to disease or, in particular areas, problems of genetic disability associated with consanguineous relationships as in Middle Eastern or Semitic communities. Further, such an approach overlooks the interactive nature of causation in many, if not all conditions. It limits any concept of primary (or precipitating) and secondary causation where the secondary causation may be more damaging than the original condition. For example, a malformed lower limb, may in a developing country make it impossible for a child to receive early educational intervention because of the attitude of the parents to physical disability, or the remoteness of the child's rural environment from educational facilities (Brown, 1966).

Most, if not all, conditions of disabilities are now recognized to be systemic and the more adverse or limiting the environment, the greater the number of potentially negative factors which can intervene and interact to promote further handicap. Thus, a child within a developing country may face a greater array of negative and interacting causative factors. A female child with phenylketonuria, and born in a rural Moslem family where there are already several other children, is less likely to be identified as suffering from PKU at birth than a female child born to a Moslem family in a modern urban hospital in a developed country. In the first situation, the treatment may be delayed or non-existent partly due to lack of service, but also because of the different value attached to female compared to male offspring within the society. Yet in the first place the precipitating situation can result from marriage amongst related family members. This example indicates just three of the interacting causes. However, in developed countries there may be other factors which interact in the disabling complex. Even within such countries it tends to be the poorer and less developed communities which are often most affected by disability (Birch and Gussow, 1970). For example in Canada, Minnemata's disease was first diagnosed in rural Indian communities.

DISABILITY AS A SYSTEMIC CONDITION

It can be argued that in both developing and developed countries disability should be seen within a systemic rather than a linear model of causation. Heightened knowledge of the interacting nature of causation not only enhances identification but also increases the likelihood of intervention, and to ignore such a systemic approach can lead to acceptance of disability as an inevitable and direct consequence of living in a particular community.

Awareness of these issues amongst professionals, community workers and parents can at least reduce the increase of secondary causal variables which tend to increase as the child grows. Early awareness and early intervention is therefore important not only because it deals with existing causation, but because it reduces the accumulation of other causative factors and the likely need for later intervention. Secondary causation has been defined by Brown and Hughson (1987) as those conditions which add further disadvantage to the precipitating cause of disability and thus can be regarded as further handicap. For example, a negative community attitude to children with Down's Syndrome can be viewed as secondary handicap, because the effect is to reduce stimulation and social contact for the child and possibly increase negative self-image. Even here the argument is limited as the same secondary impacts may have differential effects. For example, a high level of psychological stimulation may produce a positive effect in some children and a negative effect in others. It would seem more appropriate to refer to impact as primary or secondary and describe the effect(s) quite separately as negative or positive. It is important at this stage to avoid labelling processes as handicapping or non-handicapping for the same social and psychological factors and probably a range of physical (including nutritional) factors have variable effects on different children.

The above argument also illustrates that there is no arbitrary distinction between disability and normal behaviour, nor is there a one-to-one relationship between adversity of environmental stimulation and disability. An interacting constellation of variables can result in individuals under-performing to differing degrees and a change in the valency of any one variable is likely to lead to the introduction of other factors, thus increasing or decreasing the level of handicap. Further, as societies change, so new precipitating and interacting causes are introduced. For example, the increase in lead waste in developed countries due to the increase in automobiles and industrial by-products or the presence of dioxin in effluent from pulp mills can represent important additional hazards in the field of disability.

The value of a systemic approach towards disability also involves the recognition of the cyclic nature of interaction — multiple causation where 'factor A' may influence 'factor B', changing it so that it in turn changes 'factor A' again. Such complexities defy a simple distinction of disability from handicap, except in the most rudimentary and concrete forms. Thus the World Programme of Action (1986) defines handicap in such a way that it may also become a disability. Although the distinction between handicap and disability has had practical uses, it also serves to confuse the nature of disability and handicap. Some degree of disability is likely to be universal. No child can yet escape the presence of some negative and disabling impacts.

But what is the value of such an encompassing view of disability? We are forced to recognize that it is necessary to look for inhibiting causes of development instead of limiting our approach to particular areas. This is not to deny the need for research workers and practitioners to specialize, but to create an awareness in the general population, particularly parents and professional workers, of the complex and wide ranging nature of disability. To concentrate on the extremes of disability means admitting that in a disadvantaged economy certain levels of disability are the norm or acceptable and will go unrecognized and untreated. This is not in the interests of pure or applied science and certainly not in the interests of the individuals involved. The concerns expressed in the United States in Public Law 99-457 clearly admit these factors in the recognition of at risk populations.

A GENERIC VIEW OF INTERACTION

Although delineation of cause and description of disability have served a purpose for some while, our understanding of intervention and assessment must now be examined in a much more complex fashion. As stated already, what is regarded as disability in one country may be different from that in other countries because of different standards of tolerance. The perceptions of society, affected by political and economic status, influence whether or not disability is recognized, and the level of under-functioning or dysfunctioning which comes to be regarded as disability. More importantly, such perception and definition influence the extent to which we recognize and are willing to intervene in specific cases. The danger, of course, is that where there are very adverse conditions, we may recognize only very severe forms of disability and provide only for those cases. This is particularly true in developing countries, but is also true of disadvantaged communities in developed countries where diverse standards exist. Mild conditions are more likely to be tolerated or accepted when associated with a low standard of living within these communities. Thus, disability and handicap are currently viewed as fluctuating phenomena associated with our own perceptions, and depend on the conditions under which they occur. Cost factors, professional availability, economic concern, and political awareness may represent critical factors determining whether or not recognition or intervention are accepted. For example, in the Gaza Strip the author is associated with a team of individuals working in the field of disability. Part of this intervention involves family intervention programmes using the Portage model to ameliorate problems of severe disability. Such intervention has proved to be an acceptable mode of behaviour because occupying authorities and others do not find this threatening. Further, from the perspective of local people, it is seen as a humane and desirable process which brings contact and enrichment, improves family functioning, and provides supports to mothers and families who have disabled children. However, an examination of the community suggests that there is high prevalence of disability and that milder forms of handicap are virtually unrecognized or undealt with by the community (Neufeldt *et al.*, 1985). Fortunately, intervention has been sufficiently successful within families, where there are disabled preschoolers, that the programme is being expanded and families with young children regardless of presence of disability are to receive service. Such a generic approach overcomes the selective impact of the disability label. But such a stance implies that improvement is possible. Using a traditional disability model it would also be correct to imply disability or handicap does exist in the average family. One of the positive outcomes of such an approach is the recognition that society's children are always susceptible to disability and even more frequently handicapping conditions.

An awareness that children need to be observed for adversity of environment in psychological, social and educational terms as well as nutritional and economic terms, alerts us to the need to provide appropriate ecological and behavioural assessment of all environments in which young children develop. Such a process is an example of the application of developments in the field of quality of life (Brown, 1988; Goode, 1988).

In some countries it is recognized that standards of living, particularly levels of nutrition, are associated with poor standards of public health and inappropriate social and educational knowledge and stimulation. The result is delayed development amongst large numbers of children.

Countries such as India have provided wide scale interventions using field-based volunteers (Kohli, 1988) working with families who have disabled children. Millions of rupees are spent to organize early intervention on a massive scale. The issues here are the raising of general standards of care and nutrition with the involvement of more effective mothering. Thus, the techniques and systems devised for working within the field of disability may have wide and generic application to virtually a total population in a country where living conditions are substandard. If health, social, psychological and education processes are below a fundamentally acceptable level, poor development is expected. There is reason to believe such adversity will result in poor physical and psychological development. It is likely that brain structure, in terms of growth of dendritic connection, will not develop adequately (Gaito, 1966; Greenough, 1976). The effects are psychological and neurological damage. Thus disability under these conditions may be more than exceptionality, it may represent normal development for that community. Indeed, growing sophistication, increase in the gross national product, and the success of basic health intervention appears to raise the level and complexity of intervention strategies. It enables society to deal with more complex disabilities and, in some cases, disabilities which are not so easily recognized. As a result a higher standard of living is achieved and quality of life is enhanced. Yet increased development of society provides new disabilities in terms of accidents (e.g. automobile injuries), pollution (e.g. industrial wastes such as PCBs, lead and mercury). Thus it behoves societies in both developing and developed communities to monitor their environments regularly and protect children from new forces of adversity.

DISABILITY AND COST EFFECTIVENESS

Many of those working in the field of disability believe that intervention can be cost effective. Although this may be true of certain mildly handicapped groups, particularly where institutionalization has been the rule of the day, the overall effect of intervention for disabling conditions is likely to increase the basic costs of service delivery. A very simple example from Gaza and the West Bank illustrates this point. The involvement of the United Nations Relief and Works Agency has reduced the amount of major illness, including cholera, poliomyelitis and other diseases, along with improvements in prenatal and natal health servics. The advent of enriched nutrition has also resulted in a higher standard of physical growth and development for young children. Intervention processes of this type have been effective and therefore represent a long-term cost saving in terms of the delivery of these particular health services. However, the impact of success on other systems is financially horrendous. Preschool and allied educational costs are likely to rise because of increased birth rate and survival of new infants. Education costs increase dramatically (UNRWA, 1982) despite the fact that education is provided on a shift system. Intervention raises the standard of living and increases the complexity and sophistication required for intervention to minimize recognized disability. Increasingly, more and more disabled persons receive rehabilitation service. More children are recognized as disabled. Lack of performance is now seen as exceptionality, whereas prior to this such disability was not subjected to specific identification, classification or remediation.

COMPLEXITY OF SOCIETY — EXAMPLE OF INCREASING DISABILITY AND MINIMIZING HANDICAP

It is often overlooked that the more complex the society, the greater the likelihood of disabilities being recognized and the greater the likelihood of new disabilities emerging. Thus the advent of reading and writing as universal aspects of education in western communities were associated with the advent of reading, writing and spelling problems amongst those who did not learn. To begin with such difficulties were not recognized. Some people were simply illiterate. As universal education was introduced, nonreaders became recognized as exceptional. Funds were not spent on intervention. This eventually started to occur through specialized and private clinics. Then the concept of learning disability was recognized and specialized services began to develop, but on an *ad hoc* and unsystematic basis, with contradictory theories about the origins of the condition(s) and the multiple means of recognition. It is likely that particular strategies will prevail eventually as they are shown to be effective. Thus learning disabilities will not be reduced but the associated handicap will. In this context it is worth noting that initially such disabilities as learning disabilities are observed in older children but as knowledge increases, so assessment and intervention are directed to young (i.e. preschool) children (Samuels *et al.*, 1989).

At various stages a society may ignore or bypass a particular disability. For example the employment of rubella vaccination could eventually mean the removal of a class of disability. Then, the fact that some children would have been particularly susceptible to rubella is no longer relevant. Again, children who suffered delays in speaking were, in the past, often not looked upon as disadvantaged or disabled. A wait-and-see approach was often taken and indeed language delays were often not recognized as such. Increasing knowledge has resulted in the recognition of a plethora of potential hazards to normal language development.

With early recognition, treatment frequently became a possibility. But the effect of this is to ensure an increased prevalence rate of disability. Sometimes normal variations in development rate, if slow, become seen as disabilities. Thus greater professional skill in the field of disability may result in over-inclusion of young children into the disabled population.

The same phenomenon will begin to develop in the area of emotional disturbance. The literature suggests that emotional disability tends to be increasingly recognized with increase in age. At present greater scientific appraisal is being given to middle childhood (7–12 years) whereas previously it has tended to be centered on the teenage years (Chazan, 1989). This development will probably be followed by greater concentration on emotional disability in the preschool years. In developed countries the likelihood of such a development is enhanced as problems emerge within single parent families where traditional supports are lacking and also as more and more children go to kindergarten and preschool environments. At the macro level this has already commenced with the development of specialized early intervention programmes and the review of preschool environments (Johnson and Dineer, 1981). But again, with the development of new services, so new handicaps arise. For example, many of the problems associated with quality daycare in Canada (Johnson and Dineer) result from institutionalization effects. Such effects are well known in the field of mental handicap and attempts are now made to avoid such pitfalls. However, the knowledge and experience have not been applied to new domains where normal children may become the subject of handicap (Brown, 1988). Thus disability to a large degree is an aspect of societal development and is partly contingent on society's need for performance.

This perhaps suggests, that any concept of disability is limited since it must be ever changing and its degree of use is dependent on a variety of social, economic, psychological and biological factors. The more complex a society, the greater the demands made on individuals, therefore the greater the likelihood of finding thresholds for disability in its members.

THE CONCEPT OF VARIABILITY

Although it may be important to retain a concept of disability for practical purposes it may be wise to set this within the context of variability. Variability is recognized as a major aspect of all human performance. Psychologists have tended to provide normative tables and graphs of average performance and while also providing measures of dispersion, have largely ignored for practical purposes the degree of variation between individuals and the variation within any one individual over time. Little attention is paid to the varied nature of growth in terms of its spurts, declines and plateaus, but rather attention has been paid to average development within particular age groups of children or adults. The work of Brown and Hughson (1987), and earlier, Gunzburg (1968) suggest that the more extreme a person's performance the greater is the likelihood of variability amongst individuals with such extreme scores. For example, a classification of severe subnormality using intelligence quotients show that there is enormous variability amongst severely mentally handicapped persons in a wide range of simple social competence skills – some of the children learning skills very slowly and others very rapidly. The variation is much greater than amongst non-disabled children. Some children with disabilities may never attain an effective performance given our current programming knowledge. But, as Brown and Hughson (1987) have indicated, a measure of cognitive ability as a measure of handicap may be artificial in the sense that variability may be associated with an interaction of the level of a particular task and the cognitive abilities of the person who attempts to perform that task. Thus if very complex early learning is put before someone of high ability, then that individual may have great difficulty or may never learn the task or system and may as a result show a wide range of behaviour which at lower ability and task levels we would describe as disability. However, failure at high ability levels is rarely seen as a disability, but in essence it has all the features of disability except that the task is recognized by society as complex. If society requires a wide range of individuals to learn the task, then education and remedial education become necessary.

It seems possible to formulate a general rule. Learning, at the edge of performance, where individuals have a task just within their range of ability, will result in a wide range of variability in learning rate (e.g. in walking, talking, specific play activities, trigonometric calculations, quadratic equations). In young children variability is known to be enormous and therefore reliability and validity of test results may be suspect. Much of this variability may be associated with experimentation, but an experimentation not set as for older children within the confines of a formal curriculum. Indeed the development of early intervention methods may reduce early childhood variability — and in terms of innovation an over-reliance in this direction may be undesirable. On the other hand, some of the techniques developed for work with very young children may result from models which have value for intervention with older children, e.g. very open play situations where children are permitted to select their own goals. This may partly be because of the intrusion of other variables such as level of motivation, previous opportunities from which to transfer experience, fatigue, personality factors, etc. Thus disability could be seen as a process which occurs in individuals with a very high level of performance when some of them run into task difficulties but society insists that they learn those skills. It is at this point that remedial services are brought into play or individuals are rejected from a particular system. Since society functions as if it is not very appropriate to label such individuals as disabled, we revert to other labels or continuum descriptors. We counsel people out of programmes or select or suggest new areas for application — vocational guidance. But in essence this is no different from disability except that its impact is amongst individuals we decide to call normal. A notion of variability recognizes that where individuals are confronted with problems which lessen or inhibit their performance, intervention needs to take place or changes in task selection should occur.

In using such a descriptor it becomes possible to lessen the negative connotation associated with disability; to recognize that variability at any level may require specialized intervention, and that where basic intervention is absent, almost all members of the community will require enrichment.

DEINSTITUTIONALIZATION

Some of the arguments described above have led to, or are consistent with, the process of deinstitutionalization of disabled persons which has taken place in many Western communities. Not only has there been a movement of people from institutions into normal communities, but referrals to institutions are dramatically reduced. It has become commonplace for many people with disabilities to remain in their normal home environments, and services for newborn and young children have frequently been increased. Many of these services have been directed towards medical and health intervention both for pregnant mothers and newborn infants. The development of services in the health domains has led to an increasing demand for community support. Although there are a wide range of organizations which provide services the need for relief services, including relief beds, has still been underdeveloped.

In the Western World many countries, including the Scandinavian Countries, the United States and Canada, have developed a philosophy of normalization (Grunewald, 1969; Nirje, 1970; Wolfensberger, 1972, 1983). Such philosophies have advocated a range of conditions for children who are handicapped which promote development and are consistent with a normal lifestyle and a normal framework for effective living conditions. At a practical level, this means the establishment of normal routines in relation to sleeping and waking and normal contact with a range of children and adults, along with sharing regular services which are available for non-handicapped children. Normalization has been accepted as a philosophy, and frequently it has been accepted by government services in terms of nomenclature, but without an appreciation of the value change which is conceptually necessary in undertaking such a change in service direction. This has often led to the belief that services should be provided in the regular community, and that handicapped people should be involved in local community systems, but without a recognition that the practical supports, which ensure that normalization takes place, are also required. The argument for governments in accepting, at a superficial level, a noncategorical approach and a normalization stance is that they are cost effective, and that the large scale institutions, and the elaborate services that would otherwise develop for disabled children can be replaced by generic services in the community, with the use of generic professionals and the employment of a wide range of volunteers. Although it is readily apparent that volunteers may be particularly useful, it is still necessary to recognize the important role of specialists in a wide range of domains. Unfortunately there is a tendency to recognize what has been referred to as the more concrete rather than the more complex and abstract levels of application (Brown and Hughson, 1987). For example, in the area of preschool environments, services meet basic physical needs but do not provide or underwrite the costs of services, such as quality staffing or the level and quality of social and behavioural stimulation (Johnson and Dineer, 1981). Although this is now being undertaken in a variety of areas, it is the training of personnel that lags far behind other areas. For example, in education and child welfare, in terms of highly skilled personnel, these fields are much behind those of medicine and allied areas. Because of concerns of this type, Wolfensberger (1983) has suggested the term social role valorization to replace the term normalization. At one level the importance of this is apparent, namely, if people with disabilities are to function effectively in society and handicap is to be lessened, the types of activities that they are involved in and the services they receive must be those which are valued by society. Selection of task, environment and personnel must all be recognized as important, and since society values certain roles because of pay, or because of perceived role in the community, then it is important for those who design, develop and design services to ensure such valorization is applied. For example, the pay for staff working with disabled children is often very much less than pay in other areas of employment.

Yet here lies a further concern because we have throughout this chapter looked at some of the ways in which change in nomenclature takes place including the development of noncategorical approaches. However, it can also be argued that such changes are merely changes in label and if the underlying value systems associated with these changes are not put into place, then no effective change in service is likely to take place.

QUALITY OF LIFE

Probably one of the most important value changes that is beginning to taking place is in our reconceptualization of the field under the phrase 'quality of life.' Within the last ten years there has been an increasing range of literature written in this domain, although it is apparent that much of it is associated with later childhood and adult disability (Parmenter, 1988; Goode, 1988; Brown *et al.*, 1989).

The importance of quality of life as a system within early childhood services relates to a recognition that the nature of environment can dramatically increase or decrease the problems associated with young children. It is also a view of quality of life studies that the consumer becomes the major definer and controller of service delivery. But young children, by their very nature, lack control of their environment. Within the field of quality of life, which has been defined as the difference between a person's needs and desires and the actual extent to which these needs and desires are met, quality of life is more easily measured and modified for disabled people who can express views clearly about their requirements and their hopes and fears (Brown et al., 1989). quality of life is relevant to all domains of functioning. The domains are well expressed by Bronfenbrenner's (1979) and Mitchell's (1986) analysis of ecology. It is important to obtain impartial information about these domains, and this underlies the importance of obtaining information from the sponsors of very young children as well as the need for objective ecological data. But very often sponsors with young handicapped children are themselves perplexed by the overwhelming situation in which they find themselves. It is therefore essential that some form of advocacy as well as a system of brokerage take place to represent the needs of children who are disabled. Further advocates must be prepared to look at all aspects of the child's environment. Such a fundamental change in perception of disability argues for a total re-examination of the environment in relation to what children experience.

The importance of quality of life relates to the broad range of areas subsumed under its title and necessitates a redirection of services away from control by professionals, and argues that the parent or advocate is put in control of needs and wishes on behalf of the child. It is the professional's responsibility to act on these concerns or requests, to improve the quality of life of the individual concerned. Obviously such situations are fraught with issues of

15

balance. Parents may not believe that a child should have particular services (and there have been important judicial cases fought over such situations: e.g. the Dawson Case, Supreme Court of British Columbia (1983). In such situations the availability of independent advocacy becomes highly relevant. In other areas it is sometimes left to the professional to convince parents that interventions is worthwhile and can be valuable for the child (Kohli, 1988). Unlike the field of adult disability where, in a large number of cases, individuals can express their own wishes, needs and requests for change, in the domain of child services it is important to develop mechanisms for recognizing children's basic needs, as well as encouraging children over time to gain increasing control over the stimulation and nature of their environment.

CONCLUSION

In this chapter the nature of disability and handicap is discussed. Although recognizing a differentiation between disability and handicap is a step which assists in isolating primary and secondary aspects of causation, it is argued that the division is to some degree too simplistic and tends to ignore the systemic nature of 'disability'.

Further disability tends to be regarded as exceptional and therefore it is perceived at different levels in developing and developed communities. Here it is suggested that disability may be the norm in some communities. Further, the nature of change in civilization means that there are no clear boundaries between disability and normality.

Such arguments stress the need to improve our knowledge, and community's recognition of the various interacting factors that reduce optimal functioning. The importance of this during early development, including uterine development is discussed.

The discussion leads to an appreciation of the importance of normalization and social valorization which can be formulated in terms of a concept of quality of life, which has ramifications for the total population and not just members who are regarded as disabled.

REFERENCES

Birch, H.G. and Gussow, J.G. (1970) *Disadvantaged Children, Health, Nutrition and School Failure*, Grune and Stratton, New York.

Bloom, B.S. (1965) *Stability and Change in Human Characteristics*, John Wiley and Sons, New York.

Bronfenbrenner, U. (1979) *The Ecology of Human Development: Experiments by Nature and Design*, Harvard University Press, Cambridge, MA.

Brown, R.I. (1966) *A Survey of Wastage Problems in Elementary Education*, Technical Seminar on Educational Wastage and School Dropouts, UNESCO, Bangkok.

Brown, R.I. (ed.) (1988) *Quality of Life for Handicapped People*, Croom Helm, London.

Brown, R.I., Bayer, M.B. and MacFarlane, C. (1989) 'Quality of Life amongst Handicapped Adults' in R.I. Brown (ed), Quality of Life for Handicapped People, Croom Helm, London.

Brown, R.I. and Hughson, E.A. (1987) *Behavioural and Social Rehabilitation and Training*, John Wiley and Sons, New York.

Chazan, M. (1989) 'Behaviour Difficulties in Middle Childhood in England and Wales,' in R.I. Brown and M. Chazan (eds), *Learning Difficulties and Educational Problems*, Detselig Enterprises, Calgary.

Clarke, A.M. and Clarke, A.D.B. (1976) 'Genetic-environment Interaction in Cognitive Development,' in A.M. Clarke and A.D.B. Clarke (eds), *Mental Deficiency The Changing Outlook*, Methuen, London.

Dobbing, J. (1975) 'Prenatal nutrition and neurological development,' in N.A. Buchwald and M.A. B. Brazier (eds.), *Brain Mechanisms in Mental Retardation*, Academic Press, Ne York.

Gaito, J. (1966) *Molecular Psychobiology: A Chemical Approach to Learning and Other Behaviour*, Charles C. Thomas, Springfield, Illinois.

Goode, David A. (1988) Discussing Quality of Life: The Process and Findings of the Work Group on Quality of Life for Persons with Disabilities, Mental Retardation Institute, A University Affiliated Program, Westchester County Medical Center in affiliation with New York Medical College, Valhalla, New York.

Greenough, W.T. (1976) 'Development and memory and the synaptic connection,' in T. Teyler (ed.), *Brain and Learning*, Greylock Publishers, Stamford, Connecticut.

Grunewald, K. (1969) *The Mentally Retarded in Sweden*, National Board of Health and Welfare, Stockholm.

Gunzburg, H.C. (1968) *Social Competence and Mental Handicap*, Bailliere, Tindall and Cassel, London.

Heber, R. and Garber, H. (1971) 'An Experiment in Prevention of
  Cultural-Familial Mental Retardation,' in D.A.A. Primrose
  (ed.), *Proceedings of the Second Congress of the International
  Association for the Scientific Study of Mental Deficiency*, Polish
  Medical Publishers, Warsaw.
Johnson, L.C. and Dineer, J. (1981) *The Kin Trade: The Day Care Crisis
  in Canada*, McGraw-Hill Ryerson, Toronto.
Kohli, T. (1988) 'Integrated Child Development Services (ICDS)
  Programmes and Quality of Life of Children,' in R.I. Brown
  (ed.), *Quality of Life For Handicapped People*, Croom Helm,
  London.
Mitchell, D. (1986) 'A Developmental Systems Approach to Planning
  and Evaluating Services for Persons with Handicaps,' in R.I.
  Brown (ed.), *Management and   Administration of Rehabilitation
  Programmes*, Croom Helm, London.
Neufeldt, A.H., Abu Ghazaleh, H., and Brown, R.I. (1985) Revised
  Master Plan: Service, Growth, and Development in Gaza,
  Palestine, for Children and Adults with Mental Handicaps,
  internal report, February, 1985.
Nirje, B. (1970) 'The normalization principle: implications and
  comments,' *Journal of Mental Subnormality*, 16, 62–70.
Parmenter, T.R. (1988) 'An Analysis of the Dimensions of Quality of
  Life for People with Physical Disabilities,' in R.I. Brown (ed.),
  Quality of Life for Handicapped People, Croom Helm, London.
Ryba, Ken (1989) 'An Ecological Perspective on Computers in Special
  Education,' in R.I. Brown and M. Chazan (eds), *Learning
  Difficulties and Educational Problems*, Detselig Enterprises,
  Calgary (in press).
Samuels, M., Tzuriel, D., and Malloy-Miller, T. (1989) 'Dynamic
  Assessment of Children with Learning Difficulties,' in R.I.
  Brown and M. Chazan (eds), *Learning Difficulties and Educational
  Problems*, Detselig Enterprises, Calgary (in press).
United Nations (1986) *Manual on the Equalization of Opportunities for
  Disabled Persons*, New York: United Nations.
UNRWA (1982) Report of the Commissioner-General of the United
  Nations Relief and Works Agency for Palestine Refugees in the
  Near East, General Assembly Official Records: Thirty-seventh
  Session, United Nations: 1982.
US Department of Education (1987) 'Early Intervention
  Program for Infants and Toddlers with Handicaps: Notice of
  Proposed Rulemaking,' Federal Register, 52, No. 222,
  November 18, Washington, DC.
Wolfensberger, W. (1972) *Normalization: The Principle of Normalization
  in Human Services*, National Institute ofMental Retardation,
  Toronto.
Wolfensberger, W. (1983) 'Social Role Valorization: A proposed new
  term for the principle of normalization,' *Mental Retardation*,
  21(6), 234–9.
Wynn , M. and Wynn, A. (1981) *The Prevention of Handicap of Early
  Pregnancy Origins*, Foundation for Education and Research in
  Child Bearing, London.

2 ADVOCACY: APPLICATIONS IN THE EARLY YEARS OF CHILDREN

G. Ronald Neufeld

INTRODUCTION

This chapter is written for concerned parents and professionals who wish to improve the availability and quality of services for children from birth to age six by using strategies or approaches commonly known as advocacy. In this chapter, advocacy is defined, an ideology or framework of beliefs and values is proposed, and a variety of advocacy approaches and activities are described. At the outset it is noted that advocacy approaches specifically designed for infants and children during early childhood are almost non-existent. For this reason, recommendations relating to infants and young children draw heavily on advocacy experience gained with adults and school-age children.

While the spotlight in this chapter is focused mainly on at-risk and handicapped children, the viewpoints and activities recommended here are appropriate for all children, in the same tradition as programs and services emanating from the special education movement since the fifties to the present have introduced as many potential benefits for so called 'normal' as handicapped children. Like special education, one of the issues that is encountered in advocacy is the integration of students with special needs into regular settings. The bias in this chapter is the integration of infants and children with special needs into the mainstream of community life and generic services.

Another major theme in this chapter takes the form of an appeal to parents and professionals to work together as partners in advocacy. It is time to lay aside petty grievances between the public and private sector, various categorical groups and different professional communities that fragment our system. Effective advocacy consists of networks of people and organizations with common concerns and shared values working together. Without these alliances we will resemble armies of ants competing for the crumbs of public resources while "dinosaurs" in the system divide the loaf.

The derivation of the term, advocacy, is from the Latin, 'ad' meaning 'to' and 'vocare' meaning to call, to vocalize for, or to give evidence. Advocacy, reflecting this Latin background is often associated with lawyers and legal action aimed at defending or pleading someone's case or more generally promoting a cause. But advocacy is more than legal action. As it is described here it involves making sure that children receive all the support that is needed for optimum growth and development without limitations imposed by institutional constraints and fragmented services. Expressed as care and concern, advocacy is as old as the human race and in most societies the family is the basic advocacy unit; not lawyers, not social workers, not infant workers nor early childhood experts. While a variety of advocacy approaches are presented here, parents and the family are recognized as central in order to move their dependent young toward independence and self-advocacy. In its broadest sense, advocacy consists of any altruistic or unselfish act born of devotion to others and aimed at their welfare. Using this inclusive definition of advocacy anyone may be identified as an advocate, whether volunteers and parents outside of the formal service system or employees inside the system.

On one end of a spectrum of advocacy approaches, citizen advocacy emphasizes one-to-one support provided by volunteers (Wolfensberger, 1973). At the other end of the spectrum, Paul (1977) contends that 'Child advocacy is a rapidly evolving social movement for children much as civil rights is for blacks and consumer advocacy is for the American buyer' (p. 3). Throughout history there are illustrations of care and concern for individuals turning into collective action on behalf of groups of individuals with common needs. Activities involving large segments of a society take on the flavour of social movements associated with minority populations that are oppressed, who have no rights or whose rights are not recognized nor protected. In successful social movements, concern sweeps like a wave over a society, immersing the population in the issues and generating sufficient public support to bring about the changes that reformers are seeking. Child labour laws that sprang from the abuse of children and liberated them from factories during the industrial revolution is one example of advocacy as a social movement. More recent illustrations of advocacy as social movements can be drawn from twentieth century labour movements with unions that were organized to promote laws and launch actions on behalf of employees versus employers. Advocacy for consumers to protect them from exploitation at the hands of large corporations is evident in the work of Ralph Nader. In another area is the work of civil rights activists; Martin Luther King's work in the United States is an example of advocacy activity that became a powerful social movement on behalf of an oppressed racial minority.

Advocacy, like a kaleidoscope with its many colours and endless combinations of shapes and sizes, runs the gamut from individuals who promote their own cause (self-advocacy) and one-to-one activity in which individuals provide support for someone else (support advocacy) to large, highly organized, complex, social movements that are aimed at bringing about broad, sweeping changes in society (system advocacy). In the same way that healthy bodies are constantly manufacturing new antibodies to combat emerging disease entities, successful advocates are called upon to create new approaches to combat sickness and changing expressions of opposition in the system. As a starting point the advocate requires a framework in the form of a set of principles or values to provide guidelines for advocacy action. An ideology for advocacy is described below

IDEOLOGY

Advocacy must be thoughtful; more thoughtful than many of the mindless programmes and interventions that we have invented to deal with people who have been disadvantaged, not through any fault of their own, but because of ways in which they have been perceived by others and Paul, Neufeld & Pelosi (1977) state that advocacy is a way of thinking about problems and interventions. An ideology, a philosophy or a theoretical model provides advocacy with the content for thinking about its own structures and strategies and for judging the system of beliefs and values that provides norms or standards for an individual or a system i.e. a political organization, to live by. Ideally, the norms or standards of a system that are inherent in its ideology, translate into individual and social attitudes and behaviour, and are reflected by the programmes and services it provides. While there should be continuity between ideology and action, we do not have to look very far to find inconsistent policy and practice. For example, a government may promote a policy of equal rights for all people and at the same time occupy a building that denies access to someone with a physical disability.

Enormous public resources are spent on health, education and welfare by our governments. But, in spite of the size, complexity and importance of human service activity, it is often very difficult to find clear statements of ideology within government or provider agencies. In some cases this may reflect lack of sophistication in planning and management on the part of leaders and officials in the system. In other cases it may be a deliberate oversight aimed at avoiding opposition and thwarting efforts at holding the system accountable. This failure on the part of governments to provide clear ideological frameworks in human services brings about confusion throughout the system with inconsistent and often conflicting patterns of service delivery.

Advocates cannot afford to be accused of similar oversights. Ideology is to advocacy what radar is to the pilot of a ship or plane. Like radar or a compass, ideology serves as a guide to establish the general direction for a programme and operates as a benchmark to monitor services and activities. While ideology does not provide guidance in every detail, it does provide a rallying point to bring back together service providers who encounter those inevitable conflicts that arise as policies based on ideology turn into practice. Ideology is a reminder that the stakes in planning and providing services for people with special needs are higher than issues such as the location of a facility or the person or professional group that provides a needed service. What follows is an ideology framed by two major tenets, individualism and ecological theory. Obviously there are many different ways to express and organize the principles embodied in this statement, i.e. the principle of normalization, but across advocacy programs they ought to be similar in spirit. This statement embodies the humanness and inalienable rights and values of children with disabilities and it places values at the center of debates concerning human rights (Paul, 1977).

FOCUS ON THE INDIVIDUAL

Since the days of country physicians and home visits the trend in human services in North America has been toward clinic or institution based programmes. Institutions and the professionals associated with them commonly pay lip service to the notion that they are responsive to the needs of individual clients, but in reality, they often fail to serve individual client needs because they conform to the preconceived framework of a professional or institutional model. In order to highlight the difference between an individualized versus a professional or institutional model, Table 1 outlines the major characteristics of four professional or institutional models; religious, legal, medical and psychological. Table 1 portrays the tendency of each model to interpret problems, shows the treatment agent, and indicates the treatment modes promoted by the model and the institution associated with it. In their proper place, each one of the models described provide valuable service. However, we lack exact procedures for matching clients and models and there are often negative consequences for people who are the targets of services misapplied. It should be noted that there is a tendency within each model in Table 1 to define the clients problems in their terms and require that the client fit their preconceived solutions. Second, it is common for the client to own the perceived problem. The person with the special need is the problem while the professionals are 'saviours' with their tailored solutions to 'pray away', 'punish away', 'cure away' or 'train away' the problems that belong to the client.

Table 2.1: Professional institutional models

MODEL	CENTRAL PROBLEM	PROFESSIONAL ENTITY OR PRINCIPAL TREATMENT AGENT	TREATMENT MODALITIES	INSTITUTIONS
religious	moral, sin wrong-doing	clergyman priests, etc.	exorcism prayer	churches temples
legal	moral law-breakers criminals	police lawyers judges	punishment	jails courts
medical	illness patient	doctors nurses	drugs psycho-therapy psycho-surgery	hospitals clinics
psychological (behaviourism)	incompetence	psychologist educator	training education	churches

Paul (1977) referring to emotionally disturbed children writes that:

> We have most often acted as if the 'trouble' is the exclusive property of the child. Scientists have tried to locate its roots at various times in any one of a combination of substructures of the child. The problem has been reduced to the physiological substructure, the neurological substructure, and even the chemical substructure. (p. 13)

A major tenet of an advocacy ideology stands in stark contrast to the profession or institution centered models shown in Table 1 in which the client is a commodity. From an advocacy perspective services are shaped to conform to individual need not according to the dictates of a model. A tendency of professional models is to assign labels to clients and the negative effects of labels are well known. Among the damaging effects of labels is stereotyping in which individual identities are lost and personal characteristics are overpowered by expectations associated with labels. In contrast, an advocacy viewpoint rejects labels and accepts broad tolerance boundaries for individual differences. At the same time, advocacy promotes the provision of services based on individual need not based on stereotypes associated with labels. In advocacy, unlike a clinical model, issues in 'treatment' do not focus on the notion of 'curable' or 'incurable' or a learning model that is preoccupied with 'remedial' or 'irremedial' (Mercer, 1973). This is not to say that persons with 'disabilities' or 'handicaps' do not require special services. Certain conditions or behaviours may be troublesome and require interventions. However, it is possible that the trouble may be located in the social or educational setting i.e. faulty expectations for an individual. In this case intervention should be aimed at components in the setting rather than at the individual. This is the position that is put forward in ecological theory as described below.

ECOLOGICAL THEORY

A second tenet for the advocacy ideology proposed here is drawn from ecological theory. It moves beyond respect for the centrality of individual need in order to determine intervention strategies and identify the relationship of an individual to his/her environment. Ecological theory has its origins in the animal kingdom where biologists have studied the interaction of animals within the ecosystems in which they live. A human ecological system is much more complex than the systems built around models described earlier. Bronfenbrenner (1979) points out that 'The ecological environment is conceived as a set of nested structures, each inside the next, like a set of Russian dolls at the innermost level is the setting containing the developing person' (p. 3). The focus is on the interaction between persons and environments and not on the individual as isolated and discrete bits of behaviour that must conform to external norms and pressure.

Traditional treatment modalities that locate problems in the individual typically focus 'treatment' on the individual in an attempt to shrink the 'deviant' behaviour into the boundaries of the social norm. An advocate would focus instead on the rigid social norm and try to extend that boundary to include or accept the individual difference of the child as one way to mitigate disturbance. This bias in favour of the individual is the unique perspective of advocacy. In the event, however, that an advocate is unable to alter the social norm, Bricker (1982) suggests another, hopefully temporary, solution when she says that: 'Perhaps the major focus in intervention is on changing the child's and/or caregiver's vulnerability to environmental effects' (p. 256). An important aspect of education and training for children and their families is to help them cope with existing realities that are, for now, beyond their control but this should never become a permanent substitute for needed social change.

ADVOCACY APPROACHES

In North America, advocacy as a mechanism of support for persons with developmental disabilities that is a distinct feature of the human service delivery system, emerged in the late 1960s and early 1970s. In Omaha, Nebraska, programmes that are characterized as external advocacy were promoted. Ideally, an external advocacy organization is independent from government and the formal delivery system. In its ideal form, external advocacy relies on volunteers to do its work and financial support is from private sources. The advocacy functions of lobbying or striving to make services accountable to clients clearly benefit when advocates are independent or free of conflicts of interest from the human service delivery system. However, it is difficult to find advocacy structures in North America that are 'conflict free' or completely without ties to government or human services. For example, the majority of North American private, non-profit agencies that work with developmentally disabled people are themselves the recipients of money from government agencies to provide direct services. From the perspective of external advocacy, government money is tainted and organizations are in a conflict of interest when they simultaneously provide direct service and advocacy. During the decade of the 70s, external advocacy programmes expanded rapidly in Canada and the United States, mainly through the national, state and provincial and local networks of private, non-profit societies that represent people with mental handicaps.

During the same period that external advocacy programmes were flourishing through private, non-profit associations, another approach characterized as internal advocacy had surfaced in another part of North America. The armature of this development was the Child Advocacy Centre in Durham, North Carolina. It consciously promoted alliances both inside and outside of the system. The Child Advocacy Centre was supported by a combination of state and federal resources and operated as a program of the University of North Carolina.

Internal advocacy, in contrast to external advocacy operates on the assumption that even with the threat of conflict of interest it is important to have the support of, and work with people who are 'inside' the system. There are people within the system that are capable of looking at services through the eyes of clients. Wherever possible, internal advocacy attempts to renew the system from within but, like external advocacy must have avenues for confronting the system and dismantling services if that is necessary. In North Carolina, the architects of internal advocacy were not preoccupied with who provided support but rather with ensuring that children obtained needed services from whomever was responsible for providing them (Pelosi & Johnson, 1974). People inside the system are acknowledged as advocates when they step outside of their formal role and job description to help someone obtain needed support. Advocacy begins and ends with a focus on the needs of individuals in contrast to system maintenance needs or staff convenience. In the literature of Paul and Neufeld there is no reference to advocacy as the exclusive domain of volunteers and people outside of the system. It is agreed that successful advocacy calls for alliances that include an array of both professionals and non-professionals and representation from both the private and public sector (Neufeld, 1974).

The position of the proponents of internal advocacy is that no one is sufficiently removed from the system to be completely free of vested interests. Furthermore, there are enormous advantages to having cooperation between people inside and outside of the system as long as they share a commitment to the basic beliefs and values inherent in an advocacy ideology.

Apart from specific references to children in the 1959 Danish legislation, child advocacy activity in North Carolina was the only advocacy program up to that time that focused specifically on the rights and needs of children. Even here, however, the major orientation was toward school-age populations, children in large residential institutions and children at risk of placement in institutions. There were few avenues for touching the lives of infants at risk and preschool children through specific advocacy programs.

Whereas the growth of external advocacy took place mostly through the private non-profit sector, internal advocacy was promoted through agencies of government. In 1975, the United States government revised its rehabilitation act (PL 91-571 as amended in 1975 by PL 94-103). The amended legislation included important revisions aimed at protection of the rights and needs of adults with developmental disabilities. State-wide planning and coordination of services and protection and advocacy provisions were important features in this act. The Division of Development Disabilities in Washington, DC drew upon the internal and system advocacy experience in North Carolina to implement programmes of advocacy in every state throughout the nation. State councils brought together consumers (people with development disabilities and / or their parents), representatives from state agencies and service providers on the assumption that these alliances are essential for effective advocacy. The agency that was responsible for conducting the protection and advocacy provision of the legislation was to be located at 'arms length' from government. The effectiveness of the internal advocacy approach described above varies from state to state. However, their contribution to advocacy activities is noteworthy in areas such as planning, promoting enabling legislation, establishing standards, monitoring services, implementing public awareness campaigns and even litigation. Few areas of human service activity in the United States have been untouched by this movement which attests to the value of internal advocacy and the power of legislation in drawing attention to important issues for people with special needs. Although this legislation was designed for adults it serves as a model for children.

At present, advocacy is a familiar term in the field of human services. Advocacy programmes are widespread and approaches are almost as varied as the services they monitor. The following Table 2 sets forth six approaches to advocacy that can be used to describe a broad range of advocacy activity. The approaches described below accept a definition of advocacy that includes both internal and external activities.

Table 2.2: Advocacy approaches

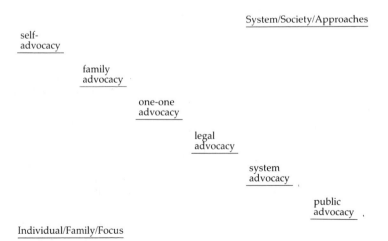

System/Society/Approaches

self-advocacy

family advocacy

one-one advocacy

legal advocacy

system advocacy

public advocacy

Individual/Family/Focus

Self-Advocacy

Self-advocacy simply refers to people with handicaps who act and speak for themselves. It is well known that both children and adults with handicaps are particularly vulnerable to overprotection and hence prolonged dependence. Infants and children with special needs are in double jeopardy. One of the most important contributions of parents to their children in the process of child rearing is to enable them to become responsibly independent. From an advocacy perspective a sound guideline for both parents and advocates is to refrain from performing tasks or functions for others that they can perform for themselves.

An organization known as People First provides us with an illustration of self-advocacy in action. In one respect it is a protest movement against overprotection by people with handicaps who resist being dependent. The message that needs to be heard is that they wish to speak for themselves and make their own decisions. In another respect, it can be viewed as the natural outcome of a developmental process in which autonomy and independence are major goals. Through the self-advocacy activities of People First, members find companionship, develop leadership skills, learn how to speak for themselves to government agencies and other service providers and insist on legitimate consumer representation on boards and committees. If there is a downside to self advocacy it lies in the realization that people with special needs have had to create their own segregated mechanism in order to assume active rather than passive roles in activities that affect their well being.

Self-advocacy is presented here as a reminder to parents, family members, advocates and professionals to avoid the temptation to over-protect, speak for, or in other ways intercede on behalf of infants and children with special needs, when they can act independently or learn to do so. Professional staff, extended family and people in the families network of support all have an obligation to work toward this end and help members of the infant's family move in this direction. A common adage in literature dealing with developmentally disabled populations is that there is dignity in risk. To allow one's children to take normal risks or undergo difficult and painful experience is easier said than done. A so-called normal child, as it matures may insis. on independence and autonomy even in the face of resistance from over-protective parents. A developmentally delayed child or even an adult may not have the strength of will or assertive skills to attain the autonomy he/she can handle. In this case, the role of advocates is to work with parents to help them 'let go' and allow their children to build the skills and self-awareness they need for autonomy. Ideally future generations of people with handicaps will not feel the need to organize self-help groups.

Family Advocacy

For the most part, the function of an advocacy programme is not to provide a direct service. Service, in this context, refers to the provision of a child's needs such as food, clothing, medical care, stimulation, etc. An advocacy approach is to make sure that the infant or child with a special need obtains support from the people or organizations that are responsible for providing the services needed. In this case advocacy is aimed at providing support for the family in order to strengthen its parenting and advocacy roles for its own children.

Traditional approaches to the provision of services for infants and children with special needs have tended to conform to a clinic or hospital model which required that the child be brought to the treatment center where professionals provided service. Contemporary trends in infant programmes emphasize support for parents to provide interventions in their own homes. More and more activities, once carried out by professions, are now carried out by parents. As early as 1974, Bronfenbrenner concluded that the most successful early intervention programmes were those that began early in life and involved the active participation of parents. More recently the opinion has been expressed that the measure of a successful infant programme is the degree to which parents are not dependent on professionals. The goal is to empower parents.

We must not, however, infer that parents with high risk or handicapped infants and children do not require support. There is a great deal of evidence to suggest that an unusual amount of stress occurs when parents learn that they have an infant with a handicapping condition. One role for advocacy is to minimize this stress.

Pilot Parents is a support programme for families with handicapped infants that was launched in 1975 by the Montreal Association for the Mentally Retarded. The programme consists of 'veteran' parents with a mentally handicapped child that have received specific training to provide counselling for new parents, make themselves available to visit new parents in their homes and whenever possible bring their own handicapped child with them. There are similarities between Pilot Parents and a project described in research reported by Minde *et al.*, (1980) concerning a self-help programme at the Hospital for Sick Children in Toronto. The focus of this programme was on premature infants that tend to receive poor parenting more often than infants born after normal gestation. This programme proposed to improve the quality of care for premature infants by their parents. It consisted of groups of up to ten parents who met for 90 to 120 minutes once per week for 7 to 12 weeks with a 'veteran mother' and a nurse co-ordinator. During early meetings, parents talked about depression, fear and guilt and commented on feeling relieved that they were not alone. At later meetings they addressed topics related to the treatment and care of their infants and concrete tasks such as getting baby-sitters, living conditions and financial needs. Parents who participated in the programme interacted more with their children and felt more competent in their caretaking role than mothers who did not attend such a group (Minde *et al.*, 1980). A significant number of parents from the programme remained in contact with each other after the groups had terminated, and have incorporated to establish similar support groups for other families.

There is certainly evidence to suggest that families under stress benefit from the support that informal networks can provide. The experience reported by Pilot Parents and the self-help programme at the Hospital for Sick Children in Toronto are promising models but they are like 'sparklers' that flare up and burn out when leadership and support that is specific to the project are gone. The question is, what can be done to create stable, visible and readily accessible networks of support when and where they are needed?

One-To-One Support

In the previous section it was pointed out that for the most part, advocacy does not include the provision of direct service. From the perspective of social obligation governments should make provisions for day care, baby-sitting and certain aspects of cognitive and social stimulus but there are some social and developmental needs of children that the formal system cannot provide even if it would. For example, the parents of children with handicaps often report that the greatest problem their children face is the lack of close friends and companions: friendships that result in invitations to the homes of friends to play, eat, or spend the night. Under ordinary circumstances children are busy laying the foundations for their own social networks when they are very young. They do this not only by gaining status with their peers but also earning the favourable attention of the parents of their peers. Because this process of network building is a subtle process during a child's early years that we know very little about, deficits in this area may go unnoticed. Parents may contribute to the problem by over-protecting a handicapped child but it is seldom viewed as a major issue during a child's early dependent years. However, the problem increases with each passing year and no one can measure the pain of parents who witness the social rejection of their children to say nothing about the indelible scars inflicted on the self-esteem of a child.

Two advocacy programmes deserve reference here and even though they were not designed with the specific needs of infants in mind, they may serve as useful models. Citizen Advocacy and Extend-A-Family are described below.

The needs for one-to-one relationships reported above fit Wolfensberger's definition of expressive needs; a role for citizen advocates. Wolfensberger and Zauha (1973) described expressive needs as 'meeting a person's need for relationship, communication, warmth, attention, love and emotional support' (p. 262). A citizen advocate is:

> a competent citizen volunteer representing, as if
> they were his own, the interests of another citizen
> who is impaired in his instrumental competency,
> unmet and which are likely to remain unmet with-
> out special intervention. (p. 262)

In the 'expressive' domain, advocates are encouraged to establish one-to-one friendships with their protégés and work, as necessary, with parents to help them overcome inclinations to over-protect their children. Typically, citizen advocates and their protégés are peers. The question is, how can this model be adapted to promote friendships for at-risk infants?

An approach entitled Extend-A-Family perhaps comes closer to meeting the expressive needs of children than Citizen Advocacy. The purpose of this program is to match families with handicapped children with 'host' families that have only "normal" children. Host families are recruited from churches, synagogues, schools and other community organizations and then carefully matched with another family. Host families invite the child with a special need to spend time at their home without the parents present. This provides some free time for parents while the child benefits from the social development that takes place in a new setting with new faces. Hopefully it is a starting point toward building the child's own social network. At another level, it is a sad commentary on social attitudes in North America that it should be necessary to 'engineer' social relationships in an effort to help people with special needs experience meaningful involvement. In response to the desperate need for meaningful one-to-one relationships, programmes such as Citizen Advocacy and Extend-A-Family may provide a starting point. With increased integration and the visible participation of children with special needs in day-to-day community activities, it is hope that future generations will experience integration to include meaningful personal relationships without prejudice to people with special needs.

Legal Advocacy

The fourth step in the phases of advocacy described in Table 2 is legal advocacy. It marks the boundary between advocacy approaches aimed at individuals and family and system advocacy. Legal advocacy poses a threat to bureaucrats and service providers and even many advocates treat it as a measure of last resort due to the cost, complexity and contentious nature of legal procedures. Despite this resistance legal advocacy was particularly active during the 1970s and registered remarkable gains for people with developmental disabilities through both litigation and legislation.

Litigation involves carrying on a legal process in the courts by judicial process. Edward Stutman (1978), like most lawyers, argues that an advocacy movement cannot be successful without it. It is power or the driving force that will result in bringing about needed changes for people with developmental disabilities. An advocate, backed by the threat of litigation negotiates for rights and needs with a 'gun on the table'. Stutman goes on to report five reasons for litigation. First, litigation is used to change rules i.e. to change a rule that excludes persons with mental handicaps from education. Second, litigation is used as a forum to articulate ideas. For example, in cases aimed at right to treatment and depopulating institutions (i.e. Willowbrook in New York) panels of experts were created to guide the process. These panels developed many ideas for programmes and services to accomplish their goals. Third, court rooms have been used successfully to focus attention on a problem. The media is particularly curious about action in the courts and television often transforms the court room into a stage. Fourth, unlike legislatures, courts must deal with principles and based on uncompromised principles, equal rights for people with handicaps have been established in the courts. Finally, court rooms have served as settings in which the worth of clients has been established. For example, the courts have won the right for children with serious life threatening disabilities to receive life saving medical treatment despite pressure from parents to deny treatment (Stutman, 1978).

The vigour of legal advocacy during the 1970s is illustrated by an analysis of litigation that took place in the United States for the five year period from 1971 to 1976. The first class action lawsuit regarding the rights of people with handicaps was filed in 1971. During the next five years, 200 cases were conducted at all levels of the courts; local, state and federal. Approximately 95% of these cases were won (Burgdorf, 1976). This record attests to the success of legal intervention. It is unusual when a case is lost.

The second dimension of legal advocacy is legislation which involves the exercise of power to make or enact laws. The leadership of Niels Bank-Mikkelsen, who was head of the Danish National Service for the Mentally Retarded in 1959, provided us with one of the earliest models of legislation that incorporated the principles of normalization and in that legislation made specific reference to children.

> The purpose of a modern service for the mentally retarded is to 'normalize' their lives. For children, normalization means living in their natural surroundings, playing, going to Kindergartens and schools, etc. (Bank-Mikkelsen, 1969)

The act included provisions for parents to keep their children at home with support in the form of counselling, child care, babysitting, homemaker services and financial aid if necessary. It called for regional centers where support was available from multidisciplinary teams in order to treat clients with multiple handicaps. These services were entirely financed by the national government.

With support from the Swedish Association for Retarded Children, legislation similar to the Danish Act was passed in Sweden in 1968. It was hailed as a Bill of Rights for the mentally retarded stressing that services should be given to each retarded person according to his or her personal needs. For children it included day centers and provisions for parents to keep their children at home. Preschool training was available along with in-home services (Nirje, 1969).

In 1975, the United States government passed an important piece of legislation with a focus on school age children. It was entitled the Education for All Handicapped Children Act and required all states by September 1, 1978 to provide a free appropriate education for all handicapped children between the ages of three and 18. This Act included the following six major provisions:

> Zero reject. *ALL* children with handicaps must be provided a free and appropriate education.
> *Nondiscriminatory education.* Testing must be appropriate to a child's cultural and linguistic background.
> *Individualized Education Plan.* Written plans must be developed for every student receiving services.
> *Least-restrictive environment.* Handicapped children are to be educated as close to regular classrooms as feasible for each child.

Due process. Due process refers to a set of procedures to ensure the fairness of educational
decisions.
Parental participation. Parents must be allowed to
participate in planning for their handicapped child
and have access to their records. (Kirk and
Gallagher, 1986)

In the United States it is doubtful that the Education for All
Handicapped Children Act would exist in the absence of litigation.
Litigation took the form of a number of class action suits that
evolved, in some cases, from exposés by the media of cases of
neglect and abuse. Rulings by the courts in these class actions
applied to all members of the class to which a person belongs i.e.
mentally retarded and developmentally disabled citizens, and
evidence from these rulings coupled with lobbying and expert
witness was the persuasion needed by Congress to enact legislation.

However, it was not until October of 1986 with the enactment
of PL 99-457 that legislative provisions were made in the United
States for all handicapped children. This act made provision for
the development of a system of comprehensive services for birth
through five year old children, handicapped or at-risk, and their
families. Services mandated in the legislation made provision for
the development of a system of comprehensive services for birth
through five year old children, handicapped or at-risk, and their
families. Services mandated in the legislation include a multidisciplinary assessment, a written individualized family service plan
and a wide range of services as needed to meet the developmental
needs of the child. These services may include
  • special education
  • occupational therapy
  • physical therapy
  • psychological services
  • parent and family training and counselling
  • medical services for diagnostic purposes
  • health services needed to enable the child to benefit
  • from other early intervention services
  • case management
These services are mandated at no cost to parents.

The process used to bring about this legislation does not reflect the same litany of exposés and litigation that brought about the Developmentally Disabled Assistance and Bill of Rights Act and the Education for All Handicapped Children Act, but it is unlikely that this new legislation would have been passed without the history of legal advocacy that prompted earlier legislation.

Through lobbying and litigation the rules have been changed. The passage of legislation, however, does not guarantee improved services. Gilhool (1978) comments that in the US, Congress has shown itself to be both responsive and knowledgeable about the explosion of rights at the hands of the court and the assertion of rights by disabled persons themselves.

> At this point what is wanting is not a declaration of rights, what is wanting is their reality. Rights we have in abundance. A civil reality we have yet to create. That is your central opportunity and burden. (Gilhool, 1978)

For advocates in countries like Denmark, Sweden and the United States where there is specific legislation for infants and other preschool children, their task is to familiarize themselves with the legislation, identify areas of responsibility within the system for providing services and then setting up accountability mechanisms to ensure that the services are provided. Elsewhere in the world, legislation in places like Denmark, Sweden and the United States can serve as models to promote and implement programmes that respond to the full range of individual human and legal rights of children with developmental disabilities.

System Advocacy

System refers generally to an organization, consisting of more than one body, in which the members of that organization work together toward a common purpose. In this context the focus is on the human service system which is made up of agencies that have been set up to serve the basic medical, social, educational and welfare needs of a specific geographic or political constituency.

Wolfensberger and Zauha (1973) do not use the term system advocacy use several terms that have similar connotations such as collective advocacy, corporate advocacy, class advocacy and group advocacy. They define collective advocacy as:

> ...individuals who work together as a group to represent the interests of another group of individuals. Similar to corporate advocacy, the representation of interests extends from group to group and generally is not extensively concerned with individuals. (p. 262)

Eklund (1976) offers a working definition of system advocacy which states that it is 'the process of influencing social and political systems to bring about change for groups of people'. According to Weingold (1977):

> ...system advocacy consists of those activities aimed not at ameliorating a single situation but at changing the entire legal framework under which such situations may arise. In other words, system advocacy means changing society — its laws, regulations, service delivery systems, customs, or attitudes — to create a climate for the development of services as a matter of right for developmentally disabled persons. (p. 190).

Organizations that focus attention on system advocacy activities include both internal and external mechanisms. Externally, private, non-profit voluntary societies are particularly valuable in lobbying and providing 'muscle' when inflexible bureaucracies fail to respond to negotiation and confrontation is needed. The limitations of advocacy originating from voluntary associations is rooted in suspicion and hostility between the public sector (professionals and civil servants) and the private sector (consumers and parents). These negative attitudes often result in counter productive activities.

The potential of professional organizations as effective advocacy mechanisms is suspect because they may be or are perceived to be preoccupied with the self-seeking interests and well-being of staff and maintaining the status quo of the system versus the legitimate rights and needs of their developmentally disabled clients. In contrast to this perception, there are examples of professional organizations that devote extensive time and resources to further the cause of their clients. One such organization is the Council for Exceptional Children (CEC) whose membership consists mainly of teachers who serve children with special needs. CEC played an important role in lobbying for the passage of the US Education for All Handicapped Children Act (PL 94-142) in 1975. Within the framework of the educational system there are many selfless and dedicated teachers in local schools who move far beyond formal system requirements and job descriptions to improve the quality of life and educational opportunities for students. Surely this qualifies as advocacy.

Another system advocacy model that had its origins in the Scandanavian countries is the Ombudsman. When investigations highlight flaws in the system, efforts are made to remedy these flaws to prevent repetitions of the problem. The Scandanavian concept of Ombudsman is increasingly being implemented and, where necessary, adapted in other jurisdictions. The limitations of the Ombudsman concept are those that apply to all internal advocacy organizations; the risk of control or co-optation by the government that supports it. Only public pressure on government officials and support from external advocacy organizations can prevent the 'handcuffs' and 'hobbles' that governments are tempted to place on the Ombudsman role.

Examples of system advocacy activities include the promotion of legislation to protect the rights and needs of people with developmental disabilities, the development of standards for facilities and services, monitoring the quality of services and the implementation of public awareness campaigns. Experience teaches us that system advocacy is most effective when internal and external advocates work together.

What issues does system advocacy as described above raise for people involved with at-risk infants and children? An important issue is that the new generation of parents with at-risk infants are not 'joiners' of special interest groups. The reasons are not fully known. Using associations of the mentally handicapped as an example, they tend to focus mainly on issues relating to older populations. The majority of their members are parents who started the associations in the 1950s and 1960s and whose children are now adults. Second, the parents of infants and young children are often overwhelmed with new family responsibility and have limited time for activities outside of the home. Third, they may not see a relationship between involvement in system advocacy and day-to-day services for their children. The effect of this low level of involvement is clear — there is very little system advocacy activity from the private sector that focuses specifically on infants and children. Also there is lack of continuity in action and services from one age group of infants to the next. In five short years the parents move rapidly from one set of concerns to another as their children grow. It takes time and experience to gain the skills and sophistication required to deal with 'the system'. Apart from isolated pockets of advocacy activity, responsibility concerning advocacy for infants and young children has fallen mainly on the shoulders of professionals and other employees in the field. Unfortunately they are at a serious disadvantage when they operate without support from parents since the voice of professionals and employees is often discounted because they have vested interests. The solution is for parents and professionals to work together.

Public Awareness Advocacy

The final step in the stages of advocacy as portrayed in Table 2 is public advocacy but it is, in many respects, the most important of all of the stages shown. Public advocacy refers to the need for the development of widespread positive attitudes toward people with special needs. No matter which way we turn we cannot escape evidence of negative attitudes in the general population toward people with handicaps and of the detrimental effects of these attitudes on both individuals with special needs and their families. Negative attitudes show up as over-protectiveness or sometimes over-solicitous behavior, lack of friends, jokes and negative reference, exclusion from activities and environments, stereotyping and labelling and in general the lack of awareness about and sensitivity to the rights and needs of people with handicaps. In the absence of these negative public attitudes there would be no need to provide the advocacy activities recommended here, or at least no more support than is required by people everywhere. The question is, how can we turn the tide of negative public attitudes toward people with handicaps and help people everywhere develop the kind of positive attitudes between people that are needed?

Three recommendations are set forth here as follows: public awareness campaigns, exposés of abuses and neglect where needed and finally, efforts to bring people with special needs forward into public places and into regular services. The problem with public awareness campaigns is that they require special skills to develop and implement and they are expensive. Many advocates contend that they are not worth the effort and expense that they call for and admittedly, impact is difficult to determine. However, successful corporations spend enormous resources to manipulate public attitudes toward their products. If it works for them, common sense suggests that similar procedures which, if properly conducted, should work for people with special needs.

One campaign that was conducted in British Columbia, Canada, in 1980 was known as the 'My Turn Campaign'. It was a major project of the BC Broadcasters Association, backed by the British Columbia Association for the Mentally Retarded (now known as the British Columbia Association for Community Living) and implemented by a committee of four people. The committee consisted of two experts in advertising, one with a strong background in music. A third member had vast experience in radio and the fourth was a professional in the field of special education and developmental disabilities. Three of the committee had family members with mental handicaps.

The committee began its project by producing a slide tape presentation known as 'What A Life'. Most of the production costs were borne by volunteer contributors: photographers, musicians, and production staff. The message presented in the slide tape was 'up-beat' with an original music score written by one of the committee. The slide tape was presented at an annual meeting of the Provincial Broadcaster's Association and representatives from every TV and radio station in the province signed contracts to present 15–20 second spots on prime time radio and television for one year. It is estimated that approximately $1.5 – 2.0 million dollars of broadcasting was dedicated to the project and this project marked the beginning of similar social service projects that the Broadcaster's Association sponsor each year. Evidence of benefit from the programme were numerous positive comments from people who saw the spots and reported positive reactions to the messages they saw and heard. Beyond that, it was not possible to measure the impact of this approach but there was general agreement that it was worth while. A further benefit of this campaign is that representatives from the media throughout the province became more aware of issues in the field of mental retardation and became allies of the advocacy movement.

The 'My Turn Campaign' is a powerful example of an advertising project with a positive, 'up-beat' message that can make a difference and one can never measure how far the 'ripples' will spread. In a completely different direction, the media, TV, radio and the press commonly report negative information in the news. For example, journalists have produced sensational exposés of neglect and abuse of people in institutions to bring these issues to the public eye. In the United States these accounts have resulted in both litigation and legislation with the result that residents from institutions are being brought into decent and 'normalized' living facilities in the community. Reports of negative information are risky because they may not always have the desired effect of producing positive attitudes in the general public toward the subject of the reports. The effect may be pity, sympathy and even horror that reinforces the perception that people with handicaps are incapable of integration into the mainstream of society. There is risk that these messages may emphasize differences from rather than similarities to others. However, dramatic measures are sometimes necessary in order to raise the concern of public officials. The media, like litigation, is a 'gun on the table'. However, most advocates long for the day when there is no longer the need for such drastic action.

Finally, concerning public attitudes, there is evidence to support the idea that personal encounter between handicapped and non-handicapped people is the most effective way to improve attitudes toward people with special needs. If this is true it is of utmost importance that parents bring their handicapped infants into public places like mothers and fathers of so called 'normal' children and insist on integrating them into regular services of every kind. Hopefully, over time, relatives, neighbours and friends of parents that have children with special needs will join in the celebrations typically associated with new children and new parents and that today's generation of infants at-risk will greet their peers tomorrow as equals.

CONCLUSION

Reflecting on the history of advocacy as reported here progress has been made in several areas, particularly certain advocacy related functions within the system. For example, pressure from advocacy groups for accountability measures has resulted in standards and guidelines for services. Along with these standards and guidelines more and more agencies are subject to regular program audits enabling advocates to reduce the energy they devote to monitoring. It should be noted, however, that advocacy organizations cannot ignore this area completely since internal monitors need to have external advocates looking over their shoulders to make certain that compromise due to conflict of interest is avoided.

In some places, most notably the Scandinavian countries, the United States and parts of Canada, legislation has been passed providing formal guarantees for services. These measures have had the effect of shifting pressure from the shoulders of advocates to the system. Also, in most parts of the world there is increased sensitivity to, and awareness of the benefits that result from parent and/or consumer participation in decisions that affect their lives. This is reflected in consumer representation in human service organizations and participation in planning activities.

It is clear, however, that limited progress has been made at the level of personal support for individuals with special needs and support for at-risk or handicapped infants and children. Existing networks focus mainly on school-age children and adults and the new generation of parents are not 'joiners'. This suggests the need for existing associations to make concentrated efforts to serve the needs of this population and there will be long term benefits for infants and children if their parents identify with the consumer movements.

Considering lack of progress we have made in the important area of personal support it may be time to look for some new solutions. One possible solution that applies to all categories of support advocacy lies is the notion of creating a comprehensive one stop human service center located in neighbourhoods. We have come through an era in human service provision of thinking that 'big is beautiful' and that centralized control is effective and efficient. This thinking is reflected in large composite high schools, large residential institutions that house colonies of people with various conditions and giant medical complexes. Typically, state or provincial and federal agencies angle for control over services but this approach establishes a great gulf between clients and decision makers. On the professional side, we have been guilty of over-specializing without the skills to back up our claims as 'experts'.

This author defines neighbourhood as the boundaries of a local elementary school. It is recommended here as a logical setting for the placement of representatives from all social, health, welfare, and educational agencies birth to death. In this setting problems often associated with service coordination between agencies would be minimized, system planning would be manageable and responsiveness to individual needs would be less difficult. This approach would increase the likelihood of parent participation in services and reduce the rift between parents and professionals. Furthermore, a neighbourhood model is consistent with ecological theory (i.e. an individual's immediate environment), and a setting in which the principles of individualism and normalization could be readily applied. Obviously some direct services may still need to be centralized such as highly specialized, expensive medical services for people with certain low incidence conditions and serious medical problems. Other indirect services such as planning, training and monitoring could also continue as regional, state and provincial and national activities but from the base of neighborhood programmes these centralized functions would be driven by information from individual plans that are generated in local (neighbourhood) programmes. Recent innovations in communications technology make this a viable option. There are enormous political and bureaucratic barriers to implementing such a system and large scale system changes or paradigm shifts are always difficult. The kind of change proposed here would call for a broad base of support from a variety of interagency, multidisciplinary and private, non-profit alliances. Experience from system advocacy could show the way.

At an advocacy systems level, parents are urged to familiarize themselves with legislation and administrative policy that pertains to the rights of their children. Of equal importance is knowledge of services that are, or should be, available and assertive skills that parents need to present their interests. While services from professionals are valued and will always be needed, parents are urged to minimize their dependence on professionals.

Finally, for professionals in the field of at-risk infants and early childhood, a chapter from the history of special education should be avoided. Current trends in special education toward integration and the declining emphasis on labelling and special services did not come about without a struggle. It might be argued, however, that needed services for children with special needs required, as a first step, the development of a special identity for special education. Unfortunately, the process of establishing a particular identity for special education has created its own set of problems. Included in these problems is a category of professionals who are preoccupied with maintaining their particular identity and the many specialized services that now stand in the way of integrating children with special needs into regular classroom settings. This experience from special education signals a warning to leaders in the field of at-risk infants and early childhood. There is a risk in over-specializing and whenever possible specialists should turn over their responsibilities to parents and other staff in the generic system.

In the domain of advocacy, a new chapter is about to be written and there are many lessons to be learned from the past that are both negative and positive in nature. The extent of our need for advocacy activity in the future, and the degree of our effectiveness when advocacy is needed, will depend on how well parents and professionals have learned from past experience.

REFERENCES

Bank-Mikkelsen, N.E. (1969) 'A metropolitan area in Denmark: Copenhagen,' in R. Kugel & W. Wolfensberger (eds), *Changing Patterns in Residential Services for the Mentally Retarded* (pp. 227 - 254), President's Committee on Mental Retardation, Washington, DC.

Bricker, D.D. (1982), *Intervention with At-risk and Handicapped Infants: From Research to Application*, University Park Press, Baltimore.

Bronfenbrenner, U. (1974). *Is Early Intervention Effective? A Report on Longitudinal Evaluations of Preschool Programs*. Vol 2. (OHD Publication No. 74-25), Department of Health, Education and Welfare, Office of Child Development, Washington, DC.

Bronfenbrenner, U. (1979), *The Ecology of Human Development: Experiments by Nature and Design*, Harvard University Press, Cambridge, MA.

Burgdorf, M.P. (1976), 'Legal advocacy: What are its implications for section 113 of Public Law 94-103?' in L.D. Baucom and G.J. Bensburg (Eds), *Advocacy Systems for Persons with Developmental Disabilities: Context, Components and Resources* (pp. 235–239), Texas Tech University, Research and Training Center in Mental Retardation, Lubbock.

Eklund, E. (1976). 'Promoting Change Through Systems Advocacy', in L.D. Baucom and G.J. Bensberg (Eds.), *Advocacy Systems for Persons with Developmental Disabilities: Context, Components and Resources* (pp. 177–183), Texas Tech University, Research and Training Center in Mental Retardation, Lubbock.

Gilhool, T.K. (1978), 'Advocacy: Toward the Realization of Rights' in C.D. Rude and L.D. Baucom (Eds), *Implementing Protection and Advocacy Systems: Proceedings of a National Developmental Disabilities Conference* (pp. 33–41), Texas Tech University, Research and Training Center in Mental Retardation, Lubbock.

Hammer P. and Richman, G. (Eds). (1975), *A Compilation of the Developmental Disabilities Legislation, 1975 P.L. 91–517 as amended by P.L. 94–103*, Developmental Disabilities Technical Assistance System, Chapel Hill, NC.

Heatherington, M.E. (Ed), (1975), *Review of Child Development Research* (Vol. 5), University of Chicago Press, Chicago.

Kirk, S.A. and Gallagher, J.J. (1986), *Educating Exceptional Children*, Houghton Mifflin, Boston.

Mercer, J.R. (1973), *Labelling the Mentally Retarded*, University of California Press, Berkeley.

Minde, K., Shosenberg, N., Marton, P., Thompson, J., Ripley, J. and Burns, S. (1980), 'Self-help Groups in a Premature Nursery — a Controlled Evaluation', *Journal of Pediatrics*, 96, 933–940.

Neufeld, G.R. (1974), 'Council as Advocate,' in J.L. Paul, R. Wiegerink and G.R. Neufeld (Eds), *Advocacy: A role for DD Councils* (pp. 7–30), Developmental Disabilities/Technical Assistance System, Chapel Hill, NC.

Nirje, B. (1969), 'The Normalization Principle and its Human Management Implications' in R.B. Kugel and W. Wolfensberger (Eds), *Changing Patterns in Residential Services for the Mentally Retarded* (pp. 179–195), President's Committee on Mental Retardation, Washington, DC.

Paul, J.L. (1977), 'The Need for Advocacy, in J.L. Paul, G.R. Neufeld and J.W. Pelosi (Eds), *Child Advocacy Within the System* (pp. 1–10), Syracuse University Press, Syracuse, NY.

Paul, J.L, Neufeld, G.R. and Pelosi, J.W. (Eds), (1977), *Child Advocacy Within the System.*, Syracuse University Press, Syracuse, NY.

Paul, J.L., Wiegerink, R. and Neufeld, G.R. (Eds), (1975), *Advocacy: A Role for DD Councils*, University of North Carolina, Chapel Hill.

Pelosi, J.W. and Johnson. S. (1974), *To Protect and Respect: Advocacy for Your Child: A Child Advocate's Handbook.*, Learning Institute of North Carolina, Child Advocacy System Project, Durham.

Stutman, E.A. (1978), 'The Gun on the Table: Developing High-level Litigation Capability,' in C.D. Rude and L.D. Baucom (Eds), *Implementation, Protection and Advocacy Systems: Proceedings of a National Developmental Disabilities Conference* (pp.131–137), Texas Tech University, Research and Training Center in Mental Retardation, Lubbock.

Weingold, J.T. (1977), 'Some Approaches to Systems Advocacy,' in
  L.D. Baucom and G.J. Bensberg (Eds), *Advocacy Systems for
  Persons with Developmental Disabilities: Context, Components and
  Resources* (pp. 189–192), Texas Tech University, Research and
  Training Center in Mental Retardation, Lubbock.
Wolfensberger, W. (1972), *The Principles of Normalization in Human
  Services*, National Institute on Mental Retardation, Leonard
  Crainford, Toronto, Ontario.
Wolfensberger, W. and Zauha, H. (1973), *Citizen Advocacy and Protec-
  tive Services for the Impaired and Handicapped*, : National Institute
  on Mental Retardation, Toronto, Ontario.

3   THE NECESSITY OF A SELF-CRITICAL PERSPECTIVE

Len Barton

INTRODUCTION

The question of early intervention in the lives of preschool children raises several important issues, including the nature of professionalism and the role of professionals in the lives of increasing numbers of people today, particularly disabled people. More importantly, it provides an opportunity to consider the client's viewpoint, particularly in relation to questions of rights, confidentiality, privacy, decision-making and social justice.

In raising such issues, explanations for early intervention by professionals become questionable. For example, to advocate that the demand for more professional intervention is based solely on the highest of motives and the best interests of the children concerned, is both naive and misleading. Disabled people have become increasingly critical of many of the professionals involved in their lives. Indeed, they describe their relationship as one of mistrust, frustration and alienation (Oliver, 1986; Brisenden, 1986; Bishop, 1987).

Such accounts raise the question of power and power-relations between people with disabilities and professionals. The basis of professional judgment is seen as a topic of importance, one which needs to be carefully analysed and openly discussed. Thus, serious questions must be raised about how professionals define 'need' — for what purpose and with what consequence(s) for both the definer and defined? This interest on the part of disabled people is influenced by a belief that characterizing someone as 'in need', or 'special', provides a legitimization for more professional intervention. The nature and extent of professional involvement therefore becomes a topic for serious concern.

This chapter seeks to examine some of these issues and argues for a more self-critical perspective on the part of professionals, one which will hopefully lead to a more open and democratic relationship with others.

Whilst the chapter has drawn heavily upon ideas and illustrations from children and adults in school and society, an attempt is made here to draw parallels for preschool children and their parents. Indeed, it is argued that these early encounters will have a cumulative and lasting impact in their lives. The topic, therefore, demands an urgent and critical examination.

MAKING PEOPLE DEPENDENT

In contemporary society, the role of the medical, legal, welfare and educational services has become increasingly significant. People generally and people with disabilities in particular, are being encouraged to believe in the necessity of being dependent on experts for many aspects of their lives. Certain forms of knowledge, decision-making and social relationships are being given privileged positions. Institutions have been created which support the position of various professionals and these systems are characterized by a division of authority which is concerned with the nature of the content and organization of professional activities (Friedson, 1986; Brisenden, 1986).

Forms of discourse have been created that both legitimize and give expression to professional definitions and interpretations. Professionals have become gatekeepers of important resources and often control their relationships with clients through the monopoly of particular forms of knowledge. This type of professional control is alleged by Freidson (1986):

> ...to constitute a new form of domination over our
> lives, to create a new form of pervasive social con-
> trol hiding its face behind a mask of
> benevolence...(p. 1)

The degree to which an individual understands his or her rights in this process and has the informed knowledge and communicative skills that will enable him or her to exercise some control over such encounters, become issues of crucial importance. This is particularly so in the field of special education which has historically been powerfully informed by assumptions that have legitimized a pathology mentality or deficit approach to disabled people (Oliver, 1984, 1988; Abberley, 1987).

Professionals are in the business of creating 'needs' but do not always agree over such judgments. Indeed, Baldwin (1986), in a discussion of needs and needs assessment, their meaning and use across a range of services, argues that they have been used differently by various professions. An example of this can be seen in the growing concern in many countries over the question of child-abuse. Conflicting arguments have been presented over both the extent of the incidents and their causes. In England, Marcovitch (1987), a consultant paediatrician, in a brief paper entitled, 'The Judge Says I'm an Expert. But am I?', offers a cautionary note to all those who would seek to use the prevailing climate in order to give professionals more powers. He maintains that the biblical tenet, 'Seek and ye shall find', suits medicine and that it is all too easy, having made a diagnosis, to make the signs and symptoms fit. He contends that:

> Where departments of child health have appointed
> a consultant with an interest in sexual abuse, the
> same iceberg effect is manifested and identified
> cases mount tenfold within a year. (p. 13)

He urges professionals working in this field to be aware of their limitations and the extent to which the interests they serve are their own as opposed to those of their clients.

People with disabilities and their parents/caregivers are often offended by the nature of their encounters with professionals, as can be seen from the following insider-perspectives.

> Disabled people have been taught that their role in
> life is to be passive, asocial, submissive to the pro-
> fessionals making the decisions for them. (Bishop,
> 1987, p. 98)

or

> We desire a place in society, participating as equal
> members with something to say and a life to lead;
> we are demanding the right to take the same risks
> and seek the same rewards. Society disables us by
> taking away our right to make decisions on our own
> behalf, and therefore the equality we are demanding
> is rooted in the concept of control; it stems from our
> desire to be individuals who can choose for them-
> selves. People with disabilities are increasingly
> beginning to fight against structures that deprive us
> of control of, and responsibility for, ourselves, and
> hence leave us with no real chance of participation
> in society. We are the victims of a vicious circle, for
> the control that is denied the disabled individual by
> the medical profession, social services, relatives, etc.,
> conditions the individual to accept a dependent
> status in which their life only takes place by proxy,
> resulting in them being unable to visualize inde-
> pendent ways of living. (Brisenden, 1986, pp. 177f)

Whilst these are the criticisms of adults, the impact of professional involvement in their lives needs to be viewed in cumulative
terms. This includes their early childhood experiences. The
accounts we have of parents and their interactions with doctors, for
example, do help us to appreciate how conflicts and suspicions
become established very early in the life of a child. It often begins
when parents are told that their child is handicapped, how they are
told and the continual struggle involved in extracting information
from professionals. One parent who gave birth to a child described
as a 'mongol' expressed her feelings in the following manner:

> It would appear that consultants tell parents so little
> for a variety of reasons. Firstly, the medical profes-
> sion assume that a little knowledge to a lay person is
> a dangerous thing and therefore it is better to tell
> nothing at all, and failing that tell only the bare
> essentials. Secondly, I got the feeling that they

didn't think we could 'take' any more information.
Finally, although paediatricians may well be versed
in the physical problem associated with mongolism
they are concerned only with the child's physical
well-being and not with the potential of the child's
whole being. The child's body is thus conveniently
divorced, for medical purposes, from its human
social context. (Boston, 1981, p. 20)

These accounts reflect vividly the depth of the feelings that
disabled people and their parents experience with regard to those
aspects of interactions with professionals which damage their
lives, powerfully restrict their freedom, prevent their independence and assault their self-esteem.

In defining needs, professionals generate particular categories or labels. These labels can and do hurt disabled people. They
become a means of limiting our perceptions and expectations.
Thus, professional discourse is often disabilist and offensive. An
example of this can be seen in a letter which appeared in a journal
written by members of a self-advocacy group. They were offended
by the statement of an 'expert', allegedly speaking on their behalf,
who maintained, that, the move to replace the term 'mental handicap' with that of 'learning difficulties' was not in their best interests. Their response was quite clear.

The term 'mental handicap', which we regard as a
denigrating label denoting a socially disadvantaged
group into which category we have been placed,
carries with it the stereotyped image of the village
idiot and implies the idea of perpetual children,
incapable of responsibility, employment, independence, sexual feelings, marriage or parenthood."
(Charles, *et al.*, (1988, p. 12)

It is absolutely essential that we listen very carefully to what
people with disabilities are saying about their experiences or
conditions generally. If we are to combat disabilist language and
thinking, then urgent attention needs to be given to confront such
issues early in a child's life. Parents/caregivers of young children

are crucial in this process and ways must be found of using their expertise and insights in order to improve the quality of services offered and to challenge discriminatory thinking and practices. In an analysis of the past 20 years of traditional approaches in the special needs area, Thomas and Feiler (1988) contend that:

> Despite the dedication of individual workers, the planning, design and expense of certain assessment and intervention systems, in general they have all failed to achieve long-term improvements for children, their families or their teachers. (p. 14)

They conclude that the fundamental problem with existing practices is the narrowness of focus and concentration on the individual and their deficits. Reinforcing such a perspective and raising a series of additional factors, May and Hughes (1987) maintain that, on an international scale, there are three major problems which continue to restrict the quality of the services that are provided for people with mental handicaps and their families. They are the relative powerlessness of the consumers of services, the problems of organizational fragmentation and professional separatism and large welfare bureaucracies which are characterized by inflexibility and resistance to change.

These critical analyses highlight the centrality of power-relations and the very real disjunction between official rhetoric and practice, between ideology and resources. Whilst important developments have taken place in attempting to deal with some of these issues, there is no room for complacency and the struggle for change will be difficult and demanding.

SCHOOL

Little systematic research, particularly of a longitudinal nature, has been conducted into the experiences of and provisions for pre-school children. In thinking about the question of early intervention, it is important to rehearse briefly insights drawn from research and analyses concerned with the role of schools in contemporary society. It should enable us to be more cautious about accepting official interpretations and provide us with a more realistic perspective of the nature of the struggle involved if we are to see a different set of conditions and relationships with professionals established at the earliest point in a child's life. Hopefully, it will inform such struggles by reminding us of the disjunction that often exists between the formal rhetoric of an institution and the actual practices and outcomes experienced by the participants. The question of power-relationships and competing objectives between professionals and their clients will be significant in this process.

Schools are involved in a complex and contradictory process of reproducing the social relations within society. School is thus a socializing agency, seeking to shape identities, distribute particular forms of knowledge and skills and transmit dominant values and beliefs. School contributes to the creation of differential forms of consciousness and outcomes, which themselves help to sustain fundamental divisions in the wider society (Apple, 1980; Weis, 1985; Wexler, 1987). The production and application of specific categories such as 'bright', 'able', 'intelligent', 'slow', 'backward', 'stupid', become part of the central means by which notions of normality and disability get constituted through the processes of interaction within schools and classrooms (Mehan, *et al.*, 1986). An illustration of this is to be found in an article by Sapon-Shevin (1987) who discusses the concept of 'giftedness' with reference to schooling in the United States. By encouraging us to view the concept as a social construct and situating the analysis within a political context, she maintains that these children are believed to be qualitatively superior. The reifying of the concept leads to its exclusiveness and to the 'exclusivity of the policies and practices recommended'. This narrow definition and focus leads to socially divisive outcomes. It increases the advantages of those who already experience a privileged position within the school system.

In order to understand, for example, the role school and teachers play in the social construction of handicap, we need to examine the generation of categories, the assumptions on which they rest, the purposes they serve and the effects they have on particular groups of children. These categories need to be viewed not as static or eternal in their existence, but rather, as having particular form and prominence at specific historical moments.

Needs are thus relative to particular contexts. Whole enterprises have been legitimized on the basis of professional judgments. For example, in the United States, 'learning disabilities' now represents the largest special education category. Vast amounts of material and human resources are now being used in this aspect of special education. Explanations concerning its nature are mainly offered in terms of the neurological or psychological aspects of a person's makeup. Being based on the assumption that there is a measurable level of normal achievement, learning disability is perceived as an objective condition to be identified through objective assessment (Franklin, 1987; Sleeter, 1987).

However, writers like Sigmon (1987), Franklin (1987) and Carrier (1986) argue that an adequate explanation of these developments must include a consideration of wider social and political aspects of American society. They maintain that the category 'learning disability' is defined in terms of a system of education which celebrates selection, competition and that makes differentiations between pupils on the basis of individual achievement through formal testing or examinations.

It is a salutory lesson to appreciate how early in a child's school experience that stereotypes begin to be legitimated and discriminatory practices occur. In a longitudinal study of children's progress in 33 infant schools in England, for example, the researchers followed pupils from nursery to junior schools (Tizard *et al.*, 1988). They were interested in the question of attainment and why some children made more progress than others. The researchers found that ten out of 33 schools had a policy on multicultural education. Fourteen head teachers objected to the idea and in none of the schools where there was a policy had the issues been discussed with parents. Given the existence of a strong belief amongst black people that '...racism is one of the underlying causes of underachievement of ethnic minority children in schools', the practices relevant to a multicultural education are a worrying features of their findings, particularly as the researchers also noted that:

> The majority of teachers interviewed were clearly
> reluctant to see that teachers might
> discriminate,either consciously or unconsciously,
> against children. (p. 47)

Thus the question of low expectations on the part of teachers in school was seen as an important factor in the handling and performance of particular children. When teachers were asked about the issue of behaviour problems, their responses clearly indicated that:

> By far the most common cause was seen to be factors in the home, particularly relationships in the home e.g. lack of attention, and affection, or parents being over-strict. These reasons were more likely to be mentioned in the case of black than white children. (p. 133)

and also

> Children with single mothers were much more likely to be described as having behaviour problems. In the top infant school year, for example, 71% of black children with single mothers were said to have problems. (p. 133)

Comparative evidence from official reports and research have increasingly highlighted the over-representation of black and white pupils from lower socio-economic backgrounds in 'special' programmes or units. These provisions cater for children and young people who are designated as 'emotionally disturbed', have 'moderate learning difficulties', are 'disruptive', 'disturbed', and or 'disaffected.' (Tomlinson, 1981; Bash *et al.*, 1985; Williams, 1985; Lin, 1987; Galloway and Goodwin, 1987; Barnartt and Steelman, 1988; Bennett, 1988).

The overwhelming conclusion that can be derived from this material, is that 'special' forms of provision, whether they be off or on-site units, withdrawal groups or segregated forms of schools, legitimate social divisions and are an increasingly questionable form of educational experience. Indeed, from a structural viewpoint, they can be seen as safety-valves and a means of supporting the smooth functioning of the mainstream system of schooling. Thus they legitimize the sorts of ideologies and values that serve to give them their existence, (Tomlinson, 1982).

This brief overview of some of the key issues involved in the role schools and teachers play in the social construction of handicap has a number of implications for the question of early intervention. Firstly, the notions of 'children-at-risk' and 'early intervention' must not be viewed as unquestionable. They need to be understood as part of a professional discourse articulated and legitimized within social relationships that are fundamentally assymetrical in terms of choice and decision making. Secondly, the assumption, expectations, priorities and practices of professionals are not to be viewed as necessarily being in the best interests of young children or their parents. The question of people's rights or privacy can often be ignored or threatened in this process. Lastly, it is unsatisfactory to focus merely on individual needs, but rather, they must be understood within the context of a systems analysis. The overwhelming number of children and parents involved in these intervention programmes will be those who live in material conditions in which poverty, disadvantage and discriminatory practices are daily features of their lives.

It is essential therefore in any discussion concerning the question of policy and practice in relation to special educational provision, that we both acknowledge and seek to analyse the issues involved in the complex and contradictory relationship that class, race and gender factors play in this process.

'Professional – Parent Relationship'

A great deal has been written about parent–professional relationships in the field of education. Much of the material is concerned with what a proper or effectual relationship could or should be like. The form of language used in much of this material is replete with such beguiling terms as 'partnership', 'sharing' and 'cooperation'. Justification for pursuing good relations are given in terms of the benefits for all the parties involved; i.e. schools, teachers, parents and pupils (Mittler and Mittler, 1982; Cunningham and Davis, 1985).

However, we have little understanding of what 'professional–parent' relationships mean to the parties themselves. Nor do we have much insight into the question of intra-profession

relations and the power struggles involved. In seeking to understand the processes by which a child is identified as disabled, we
need to recognize that during the early stages of a child's life
medical definitions will often become powerful constraints on the
definitions parents have of their child. Parental perceptions are
shaped in interaction with others and the significance of key professionals in this process becomes crucial. Many parents of young
disabled children are unhappy with a number of features of their
relationships with professionals. These include the bluntness and
insensitivity of professionals, the seeming inability or reluctance
of professionals to give them sufficient information, professionals'
unwillingness to take parents views seriously, fears of being de-
skilled by professionals and having their self-esteem lowered and,
finally, the accessibility and role of files and records. The cumulative impact of these experiences is to create and sustain mistrust,
frustration and anger which exacerbates existing stress levels
experienced from living in a society that offers very little support
and help to such parents. (Voysey, 1975; E241, 1983; Clark, 1983;
Dyson, 1986 and Woods, 1988).

The language of 'partnership' and the reality of actual relationships and practices are often very different, and given that
many children from disadvantaged socio-economic circumstances
are, and can increasingly be seen as candidates for early intervention programmes, it is essential that we question the professional
construction of the category 'children-at-risk'. The label 'children-
at-risk' and the associated screening processes involved raise
several serious issues. For example, the label is both an administrative and catch-all one. The sheer range of possible symptoms,
behaviours, and indicators that can be subsumed within this
category is worrying. It is also at one and the same time both a
description of a condition and a justification for more professional
involvement. The issue of misidentification and the resultant
effects that this can possibly lead to, must not be underestimated.
Finally, the screening process itself tends to focus on the individual
child to the neglect of contextual and organizational factors within
the system (van Kraayenoord, 1983).

CONCLUSION

The emphasis of this chapter has been to move the focus of attention from the individual and within-the-child syndromes, to social and structural relationships and factors. From this perspective, it is crucial that examination is made of the ways in which handicap is socially constructed. Being a child means you are vulnerable. Being a child with severe learning difficulties means you are doubly disadvantaged. Living in poverty means you have an added disadvantage. Early professional intervention will often be in the home, thus the question of the invasion of privacy by people whose experiences, values and priorities are very different, becomes a major issue. Part of the problem is that few people on the receiving end of such encounters know what their rights are and many professionals lack sensitivity and good interpersonal skills (Gray 1986). Any discussion therefore of 'children-at-risk', needs to be contextualized against the stubborn reality that the vast majority of these children will be from lower socio-economic backgrounds. Their experience of life involves few opportunities or choices, but rather, one in which dependence on the decisions and directives of a range of professionals will become an increasingly significant factor.

Given the deficit-type models of thinking with regards to clients that informs a great deal of professional courses, coupled with the work context in which decisions and practices are conducted, it is very difficult for professionals to view disabled people other than in terms of their alleged inadequacies or professionally defined needs. Professional encounters involve power-relations and the maintenance of various vested-interests. One fundamental question is 'In whose interests are certain definitions, decisions and actions made?' An assumption behind this question is the desire for a particular form of professionalism, one in which it is essential to develop systematically a reflexive approach to work. This demands of the professional a critical self-awareness, one which will inform both the thinking and action in relation to disabled people and their families.

This stance both to self and others includes the following features:

1. A genuine acknowledgement of our limitations and a recognition of the fragile basis on which many of our assessments and decisions are based.
2. A recognition of the rights of disabled people and a concern to see the outworking of this in our professional relationships.
3. The need to work very hard at developing good listening skills in order that we both hear and take seriously what disabled people and their parents/caregivers say to us.
4. The need to seek constantly ways in which our professional involvement leads to the empowerment of disabled people and their parents/caregivers.

The challenge is an enormous one, but so is the urgency of the task. The stakes are very high and include people's self identity, choice and liberation. The degree of struggle this will necessitate must not be underestimated. It is one in which, as Brechin and Swain (1988) note, there are strong resistances to changing professional roles, and as they so forcefully remind us:

> The principle of normalization does not seem to translate easily into new modes of professional/ client interaction (p. 213).

The experience of people with disabilities and their parents, and particularly those with severe learning difficulties, is one of exclusion and segregation, in which a social apartheid has been established. Some of the fundamental difficulties for those pupils or young people who will be defined as 'at-risk', is that they lack a powerful voice nationally in which they can express their concerns. They have no established mechanisms for articulating their perspectives. Indeed, the categories which are used to describe them assume an inferior ability on their part.

Given the structural conditions within which definitions and practices must be understood, it is essential that we recognize that labelling 'children-at-risk' far from having positive diagnostic importance, could well lead to a form of education that legitimizes their inferiority and celebrates their second class citizenship.

SUMMARY OF MAJOR POINTS

1. Individualized models of disability are unacceptable.

2. The question of 'early intervention' needs to be set within a socio-economic and political framework. This includes issues of class, race and gender.

3. The nature of 'professionalism', the discourse and practices of professionals need to be seriously examined.

4. Issues of power and control are essential to any adequate understanding or explanation of early intervention and special needs.

5. The rights of people with disabilities and their families are crucial.

6. We must listen to people with disabilities and their parents.

7. Professionals in their relationships with young children with disabilities and their parents need to be concerned with their client's empowerment.

8. This agenda leaves no room for complacency; the struggle for change is both necessary and extremely demanding.

REFERENCES

Abberley, P. (1987) 'The Concept of Oppression and the Development of a Social Theory of Disability,' in *Disability, Handicap and Society 2*, No. 1, 5–19.
Apple, M. (1980) 'Analysing Determinations: Understanding and Evaluating the Production of Social Outcomes in Schools,' *Curriculum Inquiry*, 10, 55–76.
Baldwin, S. (1986) 'Problems with Needs — Where Theory Meets Practice,' in *Disability, Handicap and Society 1*, No. 2, 139–146.

Barnartt, S. N. and Steelman, K. (1988) 'A Comparison of Federal Laws toward Disabled and Racial/Ethnic Groups in the USA,' in *Disability, Handicap and Society, 3,* No. 1, 37–48.

Bash, L., Coulby, D.E. and Jones, C. (1985) *Urban Schooling Theory and Practice.* Holt Education, London.

Bennett, A. J. (1988) 'Gateways to Powerlessness: Incorporating Hispanic Deaf Children and Families into Formal Schooling,' in *Disability, Handicap and Society, 3,* No. 2, 119–151.

Bishop, M. (1987) 'Disabling the Able?,' *British Journal of Special Education, 14,* No. 3, 98.

Boston, S. (1981) *Will, my son. The Life and Death of a Mongol Child,* Pluto Press, London.

Brechin, A. and Swain, J. (1988) 'Professional/Client Relationships: Creating a 'Working Alliance' with People with Learning Difficulties,' *Disability, Handicap and Society, 3,* No. 3.

Brisenden, S. (1986) 'Independent Living and the Medical Model of Disability,' *Disability, Handicap and Society, 1,* No. 2, 173–178.

Carrier, J. (1986) *Learning Disability: Social Class and the Construction of Inequality in American Education,* Greenwood Press, New York.

Charles, B., Gardner, S., and McDonald, A. (1988) 'We all have Disabilities,' *Community Care, March 10th,* 12.

Clark, M. (ed) (1983) 'Special Educational Needs and Children Under Five,' *Educational Review, Occasional Papers No. 9,* University of Birmingham, Birmingham.

Cunningham, C. and Davis, H. (1985) *Working with Parents,* Open University Press, Milton Keynes.

Dyson, S. (1986) 'Professional, Mentally Handicapped Children and Confidential Files,' *Disability, Handicap and Society, 1,* No. 1, 73–88.

E241. (1983) *Eradicating Handicap.* Unit 14. Open University Press, Milton Keynes.

Franklin, B. (ed) (1987) *Disability: Dissenting Essays.* Falmer Press, Lewes.

Freeman, A. (1988) 'Parents: Dilemmas for Professionals,' *Disability, Handicap and Society 3,* No. 1, 79–86

Freidson, E. (1986) *Professional Powers: A Study of the Institutionalisation of Formal Knowledge,* University of Chicago Press, Chicago.

Galloway, D. and Goodwin, C. (1987) *The Education of Disturbing Children,* Longman, London.

Gray, S.W. (1986) 'Early Intervention for Children at Educational Risk: Some Sidelights for Learners with Severe Mental Retardation,' in P. Dokeck & R. Zanar (eds), *Ethics of Dealing with Persons with Severe Handicaps.* Paul H. Brookes, Baltimore.

ILEA (1985) 'Educational Opportunities for All?,' (*Fish Report*), ILEA, London.

Lin, W.T.C. (1987) 'The Development of Special Education in Brazil,' *Disability, Handicap and Society Vol. 2*, No. 3, 259–274.

Marcovitch, H. (1987) 'The Judge Says I'm an Expert. But am I?,' *The Guardian, 8*, No. 7, 13.

May, D. and Hughes, D. (1987) 'Organising Services for People with Mental Handicap: The Californian Experience,' *Disability, Handicap and Society, 2*, No. 3, 213–230.

Mehan, H., Hertweck, A., and Meihls, J. (1986) 'Handicapping the Handicapped: Decision Making,' in Students,' *Educational Careers*, Stanford University Press, California.

Mittler, P. and Mittler, H. (1982) *Partnership with Parents*, National Council for Special Education, Stratford-on-Avon.

Oliver, M. (1984) 'The Politics of Disability,' *Critical School Policy, No. 11*, 21–32.

Oliver, M. (1986) 'Social Policy and Disability: Some Theoretical Issues,' *Disability, Handicap and Society, 1*, No. 1, 5–18.

Oliver, M. (1988) 'The Social and Political Context of Educational Policy: The Case of Special Needs,' in L. Barton (ed.), *The Politics of Special Educational Needs*, Falmer Press, Lewes.

Sapon-Shevin, M. (1987) 'Giftedness as a Social Construct,' *Teachers College Record, 89*, No. 1, 39–53.

Sigmon, S. (1987) *Radical Analysis of Special Education*, Falmer Press, Lewes.

Sleeter, C. (1987) 'Why is There Learning Disabilities? A Critical Analysis of the Birth of the Field in its Social Context,' in T. Popkewitz (ed.), *The Formation of School Subjects*, Falmer Press, Lewes.

Thomas, G. and Feiler, A. (eds.) *Planning for Special Needs. A Whole School Approach*, Blackwell, Oxford.

Tizard, B., Blatchford, P., Burke, J., Farquhar, C., Plewis, I. (1988) *Young Children at School in the Inner City*, ILEA, London.

Tomlinson, S. (1981) *Educational Subnormality - A Study in Decision Making*, Routledge & Kegan Paul, London.

Tomlinson, S. (1982) *The Sociology of Special Education*, Routledge & Kegan Paul, London.

Van Kraayenoord, C. (1983) 'Pre-school Screening for Learning Disabilities: Is it Warranted?,' *New Zealand Journal for Educational Studies, 18*, No. 1, 48–58.

Voysey. M. (1975) *A Constant Burden. The Reconstitution of Family Life.* R.K.P. London.

Weis, L. (1985) *Between Two Worlds: Black Students in an Urban Community College*, Routledge and Kegan Paul, London.

Wexler, P. (1987) *Social Analysis of Education. After the New Sociology,* Routledge and Kegan Paul, London.

Williams, P. (ed.) (1985) *Special Education in Minority Communities,* Open University Press, Milton Keynes.

Woods. S. (1988) 'Parents: Whose Partners?,' in Barton. L. (ed.), *The Politics of Special Educational Needs,* Falmer Press. Lewes.

4 CULTURAL SENSITIVITY IN THE DESIGN AND EVALUATION OF EARLY INTERVENTION PROGRAMMES

Robert W. Heath and Paula Levin

INTRODUCTION

The consideration of culture is critical for appropriately designing and evaluating early intervention programmes serving disabled and at-risk infants and young children. It has become obvious during the past 20 years that the programme needs of children in culturally diverse families are often not well understood by those who formulate and carry out social and educational public policy (Harvey, 1977). In addition, these children have historically received services of unequal kind and degree compared with those children whose families are by social class and culture part of the mainstream of a society. In the United States, for example, disproportionately large numbers of children whose first language is not English have found themselves placed in special education classes for children with mental handicaps (Mercer, 1973; Gerry, 1973). The problems associated with disabling conditions are compounded for minority children, and doubly so for those living in poverty. The costs, emotional as well as financial, of caring for a disabled child are exacerbated by inadequate financial resources.

In the past few years, efforts have been made to increase support being provided for disabled infants and toddlers (Barnett and Escobar, 1987). In addition, the special needs of disabled children who belong to ethnic minority groups have also recently become issues addressed by educational researchers and evaluators (e.g., Bransford *et al.*, 1973; Hicks, 1982; Jordan *et al.*, 1977; special issues of *Topics in Early Childhood Special Education*, 1987; and *Exceptional Children*, 1974, 1980).

CULTURE

In part, culture consists of the understandings that people have about the way the world works, as well as the beliefs and values that are attached to these understandings. It includes those ideas that people share with fellow members of their social group, and that they learn as a consequence of growing up in that group. The most fundamental cultural beliefs are those which people learn early in life. People come to believe that these cultural ways of thinking about the world are natural, normal and true. Some of these basic beliefs concern social relationships, such as how parents ought to raise children, how children should behave toward their parents, how to be a good husband or wife, and what kind of care aged parents should expect from their children.

Societies vary in cultural beliefs about what are considered 'normal' qualities and capabilities of infants and young children and about what are held to be appropriate ways to care for children. In addition, there are cross-cultural variations in identifying and attaching meaning to imperfections in body and mind. For these reasons, issues of culture must be addressed by those who work with disabled infants and young children. In a multicultural society, people who plan policy, design programmes or provide service to disabled infants and toddlers cannot assume that their basic ideas about the meaning of disabling conditions and the meaning of intervention are shared by families served by these programmes. The following is a discussion of how cultural beliefs and attitudes about infants and young children may affect the success or even viability of programmes for disabled or at-risk children.

Crucially tied to the identification of need for, concern about or treatment of, disabled infants and young children are beliefs about what is normal developmental rate and sequence. People who do not expect very young children to be capable of taking part in 'conversations' or respond to speech until they themselves can speak are less likely to suspect that an infant is hearing impaired. Parents may be little concerned by a young child who does not babble if they hold that the distinction between preverbal and verbal is one of kind and not degree.

Groups also differ in what is identified as being a disability. What may be a disability may not be considered especially troubling or disabling in another. According to Nazzaro (1981), Native Americans are more accepting of physical differences than European Americans. Among the Navajo, for example, a hearing impaired person can perform the culturally valued profession of shepherding as well as someone who is not hearing impaired.

Cultural beliefs about the sources of disabling conditions may also affect both the recognition of special needs and the response to offered services. When parents or other family members believe that a child is disabled because of their own characteristics or behaviours, there are obvious implications for family interest and involvement in treatment opportunities. Such an attitude may lead families to reject the notion that something is wrong with a child, if the conditions are not initially overt, or to isolate the child, if the conditions are apparent. Rogow (1985) describes how service delivery within the Chinese community on the mainland United States is affected by cultural beliefs about disability. According to her account, the Chinese both fear and pity the blind. A child's blindness indicates that something is amiss within the family. Thus, she argues, sightless children are kept isolated from the larger social world for two reasons: to ensure that the child will not be taken away from the family, and to demonstrate the family's ability to care fully for all of its members. One might expect that such families decide that they must take full responsibility for the care of a child with special needs, rather than accept assistance from public agencies, since they view the child's condition as the family's 'fault'. In addition, the child may be kept from public view because the family experiences shame when others see the child, whose problems may be viewed as a physical reminder of family discord or misbehaviour.

A fatalistic attitude toward disabilities may also arouse little interest in seeking out or participating in treatment. Smith (1981) describes Hispanic parents' reactions to disabling conditions in their children. Having a disabled child is experienced as a test of strength of religious conviction. Metaphorically, it is a family's cross to bear. Within such a cultural framework, advice on how to ameliorate disabling conditions or parcel out care of the child to others may not only be of little interest, it may strike family members as a dishonorable sign of lack of faith.

Within different societies, the reaction to children's disabilities will vary across disabling conditions. Some societies, such as the United States, consider mild vision impairment to be normal, and the wearing of a prosthesis to correct this impairment, attractive. In other societies, one example being the Navajo, the wearing of any prosthetic device is ridiculed (Wakabayashi *et al.*, 1977).

The success of the delivery of early intervention programmes is obviously affected by how those who provide medical or educational services are perceived. Rogow (1985) discusses the problems which arise in providing service to a Chinese community on the United States mainland. On the one hand, the Chinese-Americans considered the professionals to be experts. Thus they should be accorded polite and respectful behaviour. But since professionals are often 'governmental officials', they are not to be trusted. On the other hand, early intervention provided by someone taking an 'auntie' or 'uncle' role will benefit from having the trust of the family, but not their respect.

Finally, as Johnson and Griffiths (1981) point out, even the identification and diagnosis of potentially disabling conditions may be confounded by different presenting symptoms in different social groups.

CULTURAL SENSITIVITY

Why do those who serve infants and young children-at-risk need to take culture into account? One reason is the real possibility of mis-diagnosis, erroneous assessment, unsuccessful programme implementation and lack of programme effect. If the goal is to design programmes that meet the needs of children-at-risk, then the first step is to assess correctly these needs. Secondly, a plan of intervention must be created which makes sense to the participants such that the implementation of the programme (or whatever form the intervention takes) is likely to occur as anticipated. If this is to happen, then a shift needs to occur, away from the notion of a fixed programme which is implemented across all clients and toward the idea of clearly conceived and agreed upon outcomes to be achieved using a variety of strategies. Which strategies are most effective depends upon the particular set of beliefs and values of the people being served, that is, their culture.

How does one take culture 'into account'? Taking culture into account may start as simple sensitivity, being aware that people differ in their ideas about the correct way to think about children. While a recognition of cultural differences is a necessary step, it is unlikely to be sufficient for providing services that people will want to use. Thus, knowing that there exist cultural differences in beliefs about how to identify a disabling condition is an important step. Knowing what these beliefs and attitudes are within the client population is also critical. Neither of these steps in and of themselves, however, does anything to bridge the resulting gap in communication or divergence in goals. While the goal of staff sensitivity to the existence of cultural differences and even their understandings of particular cultures is admirable, it is inadequate to the task of creating and maintaining a successful programme of early intervention. A better strategy is to develop programmes which are culturally responsive and culturally responsible.

CULTURALLY SENSITIVE PROGRAMME DESIGN

In order to develop an early intervention programme which consists of strategies that allow for the development of social adequacy (Harvey, 1977), it is necessary to be concerned with culture in the following dimensions:

1. programme goals and objectives
2. programme content, materials and elements
3. staff selection, training, support and roles
4. strategies for service delivery
5. language in which assessment, decision-making and treatment are done
6. strategies for child and family recruitment, assessment and placement.

Creating a culturally responsive and responsible early intervention programme, then, means considering the cultural implications of all aspects of the programme, including the process of programme design. Even among professionals who agree with the goal of cultural sensitivity in early intervention, there is some scepticism that such a task is feasible. A common criticism is that those involved in early intervention activities would have to become culture experts (or even anthropologists!) in order to know enough about the culture of the group served to make the programme sensitive to their values and beliefs. This strategy is clearly a time-consuming, ineffective way to go about delivering services to children-at-risk. There are other strategies, more efficient and effective. One is to adapt a technique widely used in early intervention activities currently, that is the use of a cross-discipline team of professionals who come together with their differing expertise to design, implement and evaluate programmes collectively. Information about the culture can make its way into programme design by widening the group of experts to include those who are knowledgeable in the culture of the client population, namely people who are members of the same social group as the children and families being served.

The inclusion of members of the group being served as part of the team to design, implement and evaluate programmes has become a required element of a number of programmes serving children-at-risk. For example, the guidelines for assessment of children set down by the Bureau of Indian Affairs (1974) state that a screening committee shall include, in addition to the health and educational professional, a bilingual person, a family advocate and may also include a native health practitioner. Other roles that community representatives can take include positions as members of community review panels, administrative and teaching positions, key informants, advisers and evaluators.

In addition to creating a multidisciplinary team which includes community members who are culture experts by virtue of their membership in the community, there are other strategies for providing culturally sensitive services to the families of children-at-risk. In screening and assessment these include multiple tests, linguistic appropriateness and a wide assessment battery. An ERIC Fact Sheet (1977) provides a comprehensive list of questions to ask in order to determine if the assessment is non-discriminatory and culturally responsive. In determining programme design, two guiding questions need to be answered: 'Is this activity culturally appropriate?' and 'Do the activities make sense to the participants?'

To make sense, a programme must have activities, goals and an organization which are meaningful, purposeful and relevant to those being served. Primary among these is the issue of language. The most culturally appropriate programme elements will be worthless unless the language of service is linguistically appropriate. Linguistic appropriateness means providing materials and services in a language and communication style that programme participants use.

In addressing the issue of staffing, it is important to consider hiring and training staff who do not hold negative stereotypes (including a deficit model of the culture of the client population), and who respect parents' perspectives and understandings of their children's needs.

PROGRAMME EVALUATION

Strategies

The field of programme evaluation, particularly in relation to programmes for infants with special needs, has undergone dramatic change in the last 20 years. The extent and nature of this change has been little understood by administrators of service agencies. Even programme designers and managers are frequently unaware of the changing trends in the strategies and models of programme evaluation.

In the past, programme evaluation was generally perceived as, and expected to be, 'summative' in nature. That is, an experiment to test the difference between programme effects on experimental and control groups was seen as the *sine qua non* for evaluation. The hypothesis to be tested was:

Is it likely (at some specified probability level) that the observed difference between experimental and control groups (on some criterion measure) would occur by chance alone, if the two groups were drawn at random from the same population.

The requirements for true experimental designs and quasi-experimental designs have been discussed widely (e.g., Campbell and Stanley, 1963).The historical roots of the experimental approach are readily apparent in the epistemological assumptions of fields such as experimental psychology, pharmocology and agriculture. The equally rigorous, non-experimental, scientific traditions of fields such as astronomy, geology and archaeology for whatever reasons, did not share in providing initial methodological direction and structure to the emerging discipline of programme evaluation.

By the mid-seventies the inadequacies of the summative experiment for programme evaluation had become apparent. For reasons of relevance, credibility and utility, practitioners of evaluation increasingly turned to other methodologies. Cronbach, in his 1980 landmark book *Toward Reform of Program Evaluation* discusses these and other issues. His crystallization of the alternatives to the summative experiment in programme evaluation provides a much better, and more complete treatment of this subject than is possible here. However, one of his major arguments is particularly relevant. In most instances, there is no question that some programmes intended to meet the needs of high-need children will exist. This issue most appropriately addressed by programme evaluation is not 'Shall we accept or reject this programme?' but rather, 'How can this programme be made (more) effective?'. This approach seeks to answer questions such as:

1. If this programme is not successful, why?
2. For whom does this programme work?
3. Under what conditions does it work?
4. How does this programme achieve its effects?
5. Are the objectives of this programme in harmony with the ideological, cultural and political interests of both the people it serves and the people whose support is necessary to maintain it?
6. Is this experimental (or demonstration) programme too expensive to replicate in general use?
7. If so, what features can be deleted with the least impact on effectiveness?

The results from truly experimental projects involving special-need children have often been ignored by practitioners. Real-life practitioners must deal with programme development in different types of communities, and must cope with many uncontrolled (non-experimental) variables, under conditions that are importantly dissimilar to those found in any single controlled experiment. The fundamental logic of experimentation requires that the results are generalizable. However, no human service programme is truly replicable, for important variations in the social context of human service programmes influence strongly the effectiveness of such programmes and contexts vary importantly.

Clearly, it is possible to employ the summative/experimental design with sensitivity to culture of the client population. However, limiting the repertoire of programme evaluation to that paradigm excludes from consideration an array of opportunities to achieve greater validity of findings through greater awareness of important cultural variables that impinge upon the programme. In addition to the broader conception of programme evaluation suggested by Cronbach, two other strands of evaluation theory have matured during the last few years. Guba (1981, 1985) has been one of the most visible and articulate spokespersons for a 'naturalistic' approach to the discipline of programme evaluation. In the serious, rigorous, pursuit of knowledge the naturalistic approach can be characterized as the historic counterpoint to the hypothetico-deductive, operationism-oriented approach. A second strand of rubrical writing concerns the types of data and measurement employed. This has been termed 'qualitative methodology'. Though many writers have contributed to this body of work, Patton (1980) has been particularly prolific (also see Miles and Huberman, 1984).

The experimental and the naturalistic approaches to the use of quantitative and qualitative methods, and the summative and formative designs should not be viewed as antithetical. Rather, they have converged to provide the programme evaluator with an enriched stock of techniques and devices. This enrichment has made the field more aware of the necessity of cultural sensitivity in programme evaluation while, at the same time, it has given the evaluator more and better means for exercising such sensitivity.

Implementation

Programme evaluators frequently serve best when they provide information, not about a programme's outcomes, but rather about how to implement the programme. This type of evaluation produces and interprets credible data about topics such as:

1. the reasons for attrition of programme participants
2. the diffusion of programme effects throughout the (often extended) family and the community
3. the acceptability of demands on parents made by the programme
4. conflicts between the values and beliefs of those served and those values and beliefs that underlie the assumptions of programme developers
5. the features of the programme that attract and bond participants to the programme
6. staff recruitment and training
7. staff burnout and turnover
8. programme flexibility to accommodate changing circumstances
9. opportunity for parent and community influence
10 the fidelity of programme operations to the programme plan.

Needs

In a non-summative programme evaluation an entire spectrum of needs assessment issues becomes visible. There is perhaps no other programme evaluation activity more sensitive to the cultural incongruence between those who design, manage, and evaluate and those who receive services. The definition of need not only predetermines the existence of the programme, but also the nature of the programme, its scope and the criteria employed to assess its effectiveness.

Needs assessment studies usually operationally define 'need' by using one of three models: 'discrepancy', 'demand', or 'dialogue'. Though many other terms are in use (normative need, comparative need, felt need, expressed need, perceived need, essential need, relative need, prescriptive need, and so forth) these three categories seem to encompass nearly all and provide a useful taxonomy for comparing models of assessment.

MODELS

The Discrepancy Model

The discrepancy model is the most widely used and cited (Kaufman and English, 1979). In this model, 'need' is defined as the discrepancy between 'what is' and 'what should be'. The distance between the 'is' state and the 'should be' state is assessed. For example, an educational needs assessment might use standardized reading test results to assess the distance between the average score of a local group of students and the mean score of a national norm group. The greater the discrepancy between these two mean scores (assuming the local group produces a lower average score) the greater the need. The performance of the national norm group is employed as the 'should be' state. Of course this leaves the definition of reading to the test publisher and the determination of the desired level of this skill to the performance of the norm sample, however inappropriate or appropriate that sample may be. If the local students perform at 'higher' level than the norm group, the assessment of need by discrepancy disappears; though it is not likely that reading instruction will be terminated.

Consider the performance of a sample of more than 200 Hawaiian and part-Hawaiian preschool children on the Caldwell Preschool Inventory. The Hawaiian preschoolers score as well, on this test as the national norm group. Yet data from a variety of other sources suggest that Hawaiian children do have special educational needs. This apparent contradiction is better understood when the nature of the national norm group is examined. These norms are based largely on preschool children in Head Start programmes who were selected for participation in that programme because they qualified as disadvantaged.

The discrepancy model involves the implicit assumption that the identification of a discrepancy (deficit) is tantamount to the identification of a need. An adult education needs assessment in the State of California (Nomos Institute, 1979) identified a distinct deficit in information about contraceptive methods in several demographic subgroups. The deficit was dramatic, though the need was not, in the over-70 age group.

Since institutions and agencies sponsor needs assessment studies, it is not surprising that the distinction between institutional need and individual need has as often been obscured. Agencies need to be needed. If the needs for the services provided by an agency or institution are indiscernible, the survival of that agency or some of its programmes is in jeopardy. An agency is rarely interested in the needs of individuals that fall beyond the range of services that agency already provides, or those it hopes to provide.

In some instances, the 'should be' condition is based on the level of service available to a reference group. For example, if children in one programme do not have specialized equipment available as part of their programme, while children in others have access to such equipment, a discrepancy may be said to exist. The discrepancy is interpreted as a need. In the absence of information establishing the efficacy of the equipment, it might be argued that no need was established for such equipment with the group that was used as the 'should be' standard.

The example illustrates defects in the discrepancy model of needs assessment. This model does not address the identification and definition of need, rather, it directs attention to the assessment of degree of discrepancy. The 'should be' state might be a statistical norm (as with standardized tests) selected by one or more experts or it might be simply some standard prescribed by an authority (as in the case of competency-based assessment). Experts do not always agree in the selection or postulation of such standards.

It is not difficult to think of circumstances that lie beyond the discrepancy model of needs assessment. It is possible to identify a clear need without the specification of a 'should be' condition. The need for food is evident without the specification of a 'should be' state. The discrepancy model is vulnerable to the imposition of the values of one group upon the lives of people in another. This cultural imperialism in needs assessment is a clear danger if anyone other than the potential client defines the 'should be' condition or decides that a discrepancy is in fact a need.

The relationship between an identified need and whatever is needed to meet that need is often more complex than it would first appear. In some instances the relationship is direct and obvious. An unusually high incidence of rubella-related handicaps in a sub-population suggests a vaccination programme. Generally, poor performance by students in Hawaii on the College Board Scholastic Aptitude Test Verbal subtest implies no such unequivocal treatment. Needs assessment, especially in education, can be performed at very different levels of specificity. The logical leap from need to treatment can be perilous.

The Demand Model

The demand model for needs assessment is sometimes employed to avoid the problem of cultural imperialism. In this model, potential clients are surveyed to elicit their 'felt needs'. Respondents are encouraged to express their needs rather than to demonstrate their deficits. Sometimes clients respond with wants when asked about their needs. Unless the survey is almost totally unstructured, the value system of the investigators is likely to influence the formulation of questions and response modes so that unanticipated needs are unlikely to be expressed. 'Felt' needs can also be assessed by documenting the frequency of requests for service, the number of people on waiting lists, or counts of clients who receive service.

The influence of fashion and fad can easily be detected in the results of demand model needs assessments. Respondents can be expected to express needs for services that are popular or those that role models and authority figures have identified as important. Less apparent, but probably no less real, is the effect of fashion on the investigators. Those who conduct needs assessment studies are likely to ask respondents about their needs for services that are currently fashionable in the professional Zeitgeist.

A number of other problems are associated with the demand model. People often want things they clearly do not need (e.g. cigarettes). Conversely, people often do not want things they manifestly need. Imagine the results of a felt needs survey of six-year-olds about dental fillings. In many situations we may truly need something (e.g. potassium) but do not know it. Respondents may be reluctant to express needs for services out of embarrassment or out of a fear of appearing dependent.

The Dialogue Model

The dialogue model has been proposed as corrective to some of the shortcomings encountered in both the discrepancy and demand models of needs assessment. In this approach a sustained interaction between the investigator(s) and the clients is fostered. Through this interaction, trust can be developed. Needs are identified with people rather than for them. Unanticipated needs can be surfaced, clarified and evaluated as both parties learn. Respondents can be made aware of potential unmet needs and can then decide on their relevance through dialogue. In this model, needs assessment becomes an active process for potential clients rather than a passive response.

Dialogue is thought to help prevent the prescription of 'higher-order' (that is institutional or societal) needs to the individual. Much programme development is obviously designed to meet the needs, not of the individual being educated, but of the society and the institutions surrounding the individual.

In authentic dialogue, a power relationship is inherent. That is, the individual has the power to disbelieve, ignore, or reject the expert's statement of need or deficit, and to reject the educator's identification of 'treatments', and views on the individual's context, values and status.

The professional has power associated with the possession of information on the status of deficits, the nature of possible treatments and their costs, side effects, and availability.

Once a deficit has been identified and authentic dialogue has been initiated, the programme developer(s), and programme clients enter into an exchange of information. To identify a need for some treatment, the clients must be aware of a deficit, must decide if that deficit is undesirable, and must believe it possible to move toward reducing the deficit. The belief that one can exercise self-interest is partly dealt with in Freire's concept of conscientizacao (1970).

EVALUATION CHALLENGES

Varieties of Effects

In the past, in the evaluation of programmes that serve at-risk young children, the focus on the summative experimental model has been accompanied by an emphasis on scores from educational and psychological tests as indicators of programme effects. Such scores have the aura of being quantitative, hard data. They also are relatively easy to obtain, can be produced quickly, and are comparatively inexpensive. However, more recently consumers of evaluation findings have recognized that long-term effects are generally more valid indicators of the consequences of programmes that serve young children. There appears to be growing evidence that short-term changes in test scores may be temporary and sometimes trivial effects (Lazar and Darlington, 1982). Parent advocacy groups, funding agencies, and policy makers are now often asking for evidence that programmes produce tangible, durable, effects on the quality of the lives of the children served. Evaluators often lack technically-adequate, culturally sensitive measures of such programme consequences. Once assessment turns to variables other than cognitive abilities, the expectations of many readers are upended and credibility is burdened. Nevertheless, good, rigorous, programme evaluation work is evident in studies that have used carefully constructed measures of variables such as:

1. parental attitudes (Andrews *et al.*, 1982)
2. home environment (Heath, Levin, and Tibbetts, 1988)
3. parental information and skills (Travers and Light, 1982)
4. parental aspirations and expectations (Lazar and Darlington, 1982)
5. behaviour ratings (Gray and Ruttle, 1980)
6. self-esteem (Slaughter, 1983)
7. independence (Travers and Light, 1982)
8. reports from other agencies (Lazar and Darlington, 1982)
9. teacher ratings

10. number of hospitalizations
11. costs and cost benefits
12. interview data from community members
13. sociogram (Ramey *et al.*, 1985)
14. case studies
15. programme monitoring data
16. classroom observation
17. staff meeting minutes
18. parental stress reduction measures
19. teenage pregnancy
20. family cohesion, communication and problem solving (Andrews *et al.*, 1982)
21. social dependency (Berreuta-Clement *et al.*, 1984).

The statistical methodology employed to analyze effects has also become more sophisticated in response to issues of cultural sensitivity. For example, one might conclude from the results of a summative experiment that if treatment A results in a significant difference on criterion B, then more A should yield more B. Yet, in different cultural settings we may in fact find varying non-linear relations between treatment and effects. In some instances, a critical mass of treatment A may be necessary before any effect (B) at all is observable. In another setting, we may find that treatment A produces effect B only up to a certain level of A and then no further effect is discernible. Thus, simple hypothesis testing must be replaced by more intensive analysis of the nature of the relationship between treatments and effects if we are to adequately understand a programme.

Programme evaluators now also have learned to look for the negative effects of programmes especially in culturally-different milieus. A summative design may show that the objectives of the programme have been achieved and that these effects exceed those found in a control group, but a broader perspective must be taken to uncover unanticipated and unwanted programme consequences. A programme may raise the test scores of a participating child, but in the process destroy family cohesiveness and set in motion a lifetime of alienation between the child and his or her social environment.

Operational Problems

In 1975, the *New Directions for Program Evaluation Series* of the Evaluation Research Society published the volume *Culture and Evaluation*. In that volume a chapter by Merryfield (1975) reported the results of a study in which 26 programme evaluators, experienced in cross-cultural settings were interviewed about their methods and problems. These interviews provide good examples of how the conduct of programme evaluation studies can run aground on insensitivity to cultural differences. Merryfield presents the following examples:

Beliefs andValues. An education project in East Africa built schools for Masai children. The children failed to attend. Buses were provided to help get the children to school. The evaluator discovered that the Masai parents '... did not want their children in school, because Western schooling conflicted with some highly regarded beliefs about work and family relationships.' Similarly, it was reported that in many cultures, gifts of money or favours were expected in exchange for access to persons or documents. Though people in the culture viewed such payment as a normal and honorable procedure for distributing wealth in an inequitable economic system, evaluators felt there was something dishonest about such 'bribes'.

Styles of Interaction. In a village survey on maternal attitudes, a programme evaluator reported that villagers were suspicious of any outsiders, that women would not interact with any unknown man, people were unaccustomed to being questioned, and that the norm in verbal interaction was to avoid direct answers and to respond indirectly to inquiries.

In another evaluation study, the results were called into question because a local consultant to the study was perceived as a homosexual, an unacceptable status in that culture.

Sense of Time. Differing perceptions of time, especially as an organizing principle, frequently confounded programme evaluators in unfamiliar cultural settings. Those accustomed to working on carefully planned and budgeted contracts and grants easily lost patience in a culture that did not view the past as something to be analyzed, thought that the present was best left unburdened with urgencies, and saw the future as something largely beyond human control. Recognizing that such views exist is difficult enough, learning how to complete an evaluation study in their context may be a daunting prospect.

Infrastructure. Local road, postal and telephone systems often made what was thought to be a simple data-collection procedure, a complex programme evaluation task. One evaluator listed the logistic problems encountered in a project to develop materials in a nutrition education programme in West Africa: 1) no ink was available in the country; 2) the printer's wife died and all work was halted; 3) political consideration prevented transferring the printing contract; 4) the rainy season began and country roads became impassable.

Language. In a literacy project, villagers were asked "What are you getting out of your literacy classes?" A frequent response translated literally to "I am learning to hold the pen." The meaning intended as "I am learning to read and write." Translation problems, taboo topics, linguistic courtesies, non-equivalent concepts and untranslatable idioms can all introduce error into the programme evaluator's data and disrupt the logistics of methodology.

Participation in Programme Evaluation

In one sense, the term 'cultural sensitivity' in programme evaluation is misdirecting. The term implies that we are going to be sensitive to them. It may well be that the only foolproof way of avoiding cultural insensitivity is to eliminate the 'we-they' relationship. Efforts to evaluate programmes that involve ethnically and culturally diverse people are best conducted by teams. These programme evaluation teams include culturally-diverse members as true peers. This will often require breaking familiar expert-client role expectations. For example the *Conference on Education and Teacher Education for Cultural Pluralism* (Hazard, 1971) makes 31 recommendations for achieving cultural pluralism in educational programmes (including programme evaluation studies). Some of these are particularly relevant to programme evaluation. In abbreviated form these are (words in parentheses ours):

1. Cultural pluralism should be recognized in the selection of personnel for decision-making bodies in all... education programmes (and evaluation studies) so that minority communities will have a policy role in such programmes. That is, no group should have the right to assume representation for another minority community in determining policy for the programme.
2. A pool of consultants on culturally pluralistic (evaluation) should be established, with its members drawn from the community, school and higher education sectors.
3. Standardized tests should be used only for purposes of instructional diagnosis and improvement of individual children, not as a basis for excluding children from normal educational experiences. In all such testing, the tester must speak the language of the child and the test(s) should be selected with consideration for the cultural setting in which the child has grown. The tests must be administered and interpreted in terms of the child's background.

4. There should be developed a screening process that local schools can apply to determine that teachers, administrators, and other educational personnel who are newly employed, or who are to receive tenure, salary increment, or other advancement, have the understanding of cultural pluralism, and the sensitivity and the commitment required to implement improved education for children of all ethnic groups.

5. School systems and universities should cooperate to provide training programmes for educational personnel (including programme evaluators) who need additional experiences in the area of cultural pluralism.

6. The need for multicultural staffing, particularly in positions of power such as those of administrators or programme coordinators (and evaluators), should be recognized in appointments and promotions of professional personnel in school systems and universities.

7. Certification agencies should develop more creative and flexible criteria for certifying teachers and other educational personnel (including evaluators), recognizing such factors as relevant life experience and a bilingual, bicultural background.

8. Certification criteria for educational personnel (including evaluators) in programmes of bilingual education should include evidence of experience in and commitment to the community (Spanish, Chinese, etc.) which the particular programme is to serve.

9. Minority group communities should have parity, along with the university and the school district, in programme planning (and evaluation) and operation of... projects... people from the community should receive pay for the services they render that is equal to the pay given to professional (credentialed) personnel of the project.

10. Each project should maintain an active policy-making board in which there is parity among community, school and university.

11. To insure that the community component has real authority at the decision-making level, project funds should go directly to community groups.

12. An evaluation (audit) of projects should be made to ensure that objectives are being met, and the results should be made public. Parents, college students, professional groups, and community leaders should participate in the evaluation.
13. Community people should be placed on the governing board and major policy-making (and evaluation) committees.
14. Projects that are funded should contain a component that is specially related to problems and issues related to cultural pluralism (in evaluation) and should present evidence of a commitment to the concept of cultural pluralism.
15. The various cultural groups in these communities should help to plan (evaluate) and implement the orientation of students and faculty to their particular cultures.
16. There should be established programmes for the preparation of university faculty and for research in the various fields of ethnic studies, including research (programme evaluation) on the cognitive structure of minority cultures.
17. Some work in ethnic studies should be required of all prospective teachers (and evaluators) and group(s) upon which such an ethnic studies programme is focused should be in control of the programme.
18. Bilingual, bicultural paraprofessionals recruited from the community should be recognized as essential components of improved education (and evaluation) for bilingual, bicultural children of the various ethnic groups.

In 1981 The Florida Consortium, a group of community mental health centres, produced *A Trust of Evaluation: A Guide for Involving Citizens in Community Mental Health Program Evaluation* (Zinober and Dinkel, 1981). This guide is a practical, step-by-step manual that should be helpful to any evaluator unfamiliar with cross-cultural team building methods. It includes recruiting of participants, staff roles, key informants, training, surveys, forums, media, complaint systems, dealing with resistance, group process skills, meeting procedures, and reporting results.

CONCLUSION

The strategies, designs and methods discussed here as avenues to better programme evaluation in cross-cultural settings will cast the evaluator in a different, and sometimes uncomfortable role. Sharing power means losing control.

To achieve technical quality, relevance and credibility, evaluators usually want all the control they can garner in the design and execution of projects. Further, increasing cultural sensitivity will almost always increase costs and require more time. Most evaluators are accustomed to managing projects that already suffer a shortage of both commodities and are reluctant to yield either. Perhaps most discomforting, programme evaluators will find themselves vulnerable. His or her motives, methods, competence and even personal worth are likely to be called into question. Indeed, evaluators may find themselves yearning for reciprocal sensitivity.

The following summarizes the majors points of this chapter:

1. The consideration of culture is critical for appropriately designing and evaluating early intervention programmes.
2. The problems associated with disabling conditions are compounded for minority children, and doubly so for those living in poverty.
3. There are marked cross-cultural variations in identifying and attaching meanings to imperfections of body and mind, in defining appropriate interventions and in perceiving professionals.
4. At the very least, programmes should be culturally sensitive; preferably they should be culturally responsive and culturally responsible. This means considering the cultural implications of all aspects of programmes, including the process of programme design.
5. Teams who design, implement and evaluate programmes should include members who are experts in the various cultures served by the programmes; preferably such members' expertise

would derive from their membership of the different cultural groups.

6. One of the prime considerations in culturally appropriate programmes is to ensure that the language of service is linguistically appropriate to those being served.

7. Summative evaluation of programmes is increasingly giving way to evaluation strategies designed to address how programmes can be made more effective – an approach which includes consideration of the question of whether the objectives of a particular programme are in harmony with the ideological, cultural and political interests of both the people it serves and the people whose support is necessary to maintain it.

8. Given the possibility of cultural incongruence between those who design, manage and evaluate and those who receive services, it is important that an appropriate model of needs assessment be employed. A 'dialogue' model, in which there is a sustained interaction between service providers and clients, is seen as being more responsive to cultural diversity than are 'discrepancy' or 'demand' models.

9. To be culturally sensitive and responsible means professionals sharing power and thus losing control and becoming vulnerable.

REFERENCES

Andrews, S. R., Blumenthal, J. B., Johnson, D. L., Kahn, A. J., Ferguson, C. J., Lasater, T. M., Malone, P. E., and Wallace, D. B. (1982) *The Skills of Mothering: A Study of Parent-child Development Centers*, Monographs of the Society for Research in Child Development 47 (6, Serial No. 198), University of Chicago Press, Chicago.

Barnett, S. and Escobar, C. (1987) 'The Economics of Early Educational Intervention: A Review,' *Review of Educational Research, 37*, 387–414.

Berreuta-Clement, J., Schweinhard, L., Barnett, W., Epstein, A., and Weikert, D. (1984) *Changed Lives: The Effects of the Perry Preschool Program on Youths Through Age 19*, Monographs of the High/Scope Educational Research Foundation, No. 8, High/Scope Press, Ypsilanti, MI.

Bransford, C., Baca, L., and Lane, K. (eds) (1973) *Cultural Diversity and the Exceptional Child, Council for Exceptional Children*, Reston, VA.

Bureau of Indian Affairs (1974) *Special Education Guidelines, Albuquerque*, New Mexico.

Campbell, D. and Stanley, J. (1963) *Experimental and Quasi-experimental Designs for Research*, Rand McNally, Chicago, IL.

Cronbach, L. and Associates. (1980) *Toward Reform of Program Evaluation*, Jossey-Bass, San Francisco.

ERIC Clearinghouse on Handicapped and Gifted Children (1977) *Special Problems of Handicapped Minority Students*, Council for Exceptional Children, Reston, VA.

Exceptional Children, 40 (8), (1974), *46* (8) (1980).

Freire, P. (1970) *Pedagogy of the Oppressed*, Seabury Press, New York.

Gerry, M. H. (1973) 'Cultural Myopia: The Need for a Corrective Lens,' *Journal of School Psychology, 11*, 307–315.

Gray, S. W. and Ruttle, K. (1980) *The Family-oriented Home Visiting Program: A Longitudinal Study*, Genetic Psychology Monographs, 102, 299–316.

Guba, E. G. (1985) *Naturalistic Inquiry*, Sage, Beverly Hills, CA.

Guba, E. G. and Lincoln, Y. S. (1981) *Effective Evaluation: Improving the Usefulness of Evaluation Results Through Responsive and Naturalistic Approaches*, Jossey-Bass, San Francisco.

Harvey, J. et al. (1977) 'Special Program Needs of the Culturally Diverse Child', in J. Jordan et al. (eds.), *Early Childhood Education for Exceptional Children*, Council for Exceptional Children, Reston, VA.

Hazard, W. R., Rivlin, H. N., and Stent, M. D. (1971) *Cultural Pluralism in Education: A Mandate for Change*, Appleton-Century Crofts, New York.

Heath, R. W., Levin, P. F., and Tibbetts, K. A. (1988) *Development of the Home Educational Environment Profile*, Center for Development of Early Education, Honolulu, HI.

Hicks, J. (1982) 'Serving Preschool Handicapped Children of Various Cultures: An Annotated Bibliography', *TADScript Number 6*, Technical Assistance Development System, Chapel Hill, NC.

Johnson, R. E. and Griffiths, V. A. (1981) 'Early Intervention with Handicapped Black Infants from Low Socio-Economic Families: Issues and Concerns', *Paper presented at the Council for Exceptional Children Conference on the Exceptional Black Child*, New Orleans.

Jordan, J. et al. (eds.) (1977) *Early Childhood Education for Exceptional Children*, Council for Exceptional Children, Reston, VA.

Kaufman, R. A. and English, F. W. (1979) *Needs Assessment: Concept and Application*, Educational Technology Publishers, Englewood Cliffs, N.J.

Lazar, I. and Darlington, R. (1982) *Lasting Effects of Early Education: A Report from the Consortium for Longitudinal Studies*. Monographs of the Society for Research in Child Development, 47(2–3, Serial No. 195).

Mercer, J. (1973) *Labeling the Mentally Retarded*, University of California, Berkeley.

Merryfield, M. M. (1975) *The Challenge of Cross-cultural Evaluation: Some Views from the Field, New Directions for Program Evaluation:* A Publication of the Evaluation Research Society, No. 25, Jossey-Bass, San Francisco.

Miles, M. B. and Huberman, A. M. (1984) *Qualitative Data Analysis: A Sourcebook of New Methods*, Sage, Beverly Hills, CA.

Nazzaro, J. (1981) 'Special Problems of Exceptional Minority Children,' in J. Nazzaro (ed.), *Culturally Diverse Exceptional Children in School*, The Council for Exceptional Children, Reston, VA.

Nomos Institute (1979) 'Needs Assessment in Higher Education: Starting up in a Small College,' *Educational Technology*, 17(11), 46–48.

Patton, M. Q. (1980) *Qualitative Evaluation Methods*, Beverly Hills, CA.

Patton, M. Q. (1985) *Culture and Evaluation, New Directions for Program Evaluation:* A Publication of the Evaluation Research Society, No. 25, Jossey-Bass, San Francisco.

Ramey, C., Bryant, D., Sparling, J., and Wasik, H. (1985) 'Project CARE: A Comparison of Two Early Intervention Strategies to Prevent Retarded Development,' *Topics in Early Childhood Special Education*, 5(12), 12–25.

Rogow, S. (1985) 'Where Services Begins: Working with Parents to Provide Early Intervention. Considerations for the Culturally Different', *Paper presented at the Annual Convention of the Council for Exceptional Children*, Anaheim, CA.

Slaughter, D. (1983) *Early Intervention and Its Effects on Maternal and Child Development*, Monographs of the Society for Research in Child Development, 48(8, Serial No. 202).

Smith, O. S. et al. (1981) 'Working with Parents of Hispanic Severely Handicapped Preschool Children,' *Paper presented at the Council for Exceptional Children Conference on the Exceptional Bilingual Child*, New Orleans.

Topics in Early Childhood Special Education, 7 (1) (1987).

Travers, J. and Light, R. (1982) *Learning from Experience: Evaluating Early Childhood Demonstration Programs*, National Academy Press, Washington, DC.

Wakabayashi, R. et al. (1977) 'Unique Problems of Handicapped Minorities,' in *The White House Conference on Handicapped Individuals*, US Government Printing Office, Washington, DC.

Zinober, J. W. and Dinkel, N. R. (1981) 'A Trust of Evaluation,' *A Guide for Involving Citizens in Community Mental Health Program Evaluation*, The Florida Consortium for Research and Evaluation, Tampa, FL.

5 EARLY INTERVENTION IN THIRD WORLD COUNTRIES

Robert Serpell and Dabie Nabuzoka

INTRODUCTION: THE CASE FOR EARLY INTERVENTION

Several important theoretical advantages can be cited for timing interventions on behalf of disabled and at-risk children as early as possible. Primary prevention implies intervention prior to onset of a condition. In addition, recent technological advances have made possible the secondary prevention of certain functional disabilities which without intervention would necessarily follow from a given organic impairment. Conspicuous examples of such advances are the prevention of intellectual disabilities by dietary correction of phenyl ketonuria or by cerebral spinal fluid shunting in cases of hydrocephaly and the supply of hearing aids (and FM transmitter microphones for the caregiver) to enable deaf children to develop speech. Behavioural techniques including physio-therapeutic exercises and conditioning procedures have also been shown to be highly efficacious with very young children. The human brain displays its greatest plasticity early in life, and any process of adaptation is likely to be cumulative so that an early start in the right direction is surely advantageous.

On the other hand, certain conditions may be self-correcting and early intervention could be wasteful, or (if, for instance, it were to promote an acceptable degree of insecurity, dependency or stigma) even counter-productive. Certain logistical difficulties also exist, which pose especially serious obstacles in Third World countries (TWCs) with a limited infrastructure of education, re-search and social services. Identification of mildly disabling conditions at an early age calls for fine-grain analysis of behaviour using precisely calibrated instruments, and generally presupposes a high level of specialized training. Moreover, access to children before the age at which their families are willing to entrust them to the care of centralized facilities such as schools or hospitals entails widespread public information and home visiting. Finally, injecting professional advice into the traditionally private domain of parent-infant relations raises, in a more acute form, philosophical issues which are still unresolved concerning the legitimacy of compulsory education.

The fact that the techniques and strategies of early assessment and intervention are still relatively new makes it all the more important for service designers in TWCs to scrutinize them closely before deciding whether they are applicable in their particular socio-cultural, political and economic circumstances and if so, how they are applicable. This chapter will not attempt to analyze the experience of industrialized countries with early intervention since this has been covered in other chapters. The focus will be on certain quite general problems of application in Third World settings.

THE POLITICS OF DISABILITY IN THIRD WORLD COUNTRIES

The majority of studies showing results of early intervention programmes have been reported from North America, Britain and Australia. Before embarking on such a programme in a Third World country, several issues need to be considered. Is the theoretical basis of programmes designed for an industrialized country valid in this new setting? Is this country's economy capable of sustaining such a programme? Is it appropriate to lay so much emphasis on a programme of this nature in a country whose economy is ailing? (Marfo and Kysela, 1983).

Indeed the question of priorities can become a stumbling block in developing services for disabled children in a TWC. Many policy makers argue that scarce resources should be directed more towards those efforts that serve the majority of the people much of the international advocacy during and since the International Year of the Disabled Person has emphasized the large numbers of children and families affected by disability, a more compelling reason for action may be the sheer severity of their needs, coupled with the feasibility of effective intervention.

If a technical case is to be made for an early, preventive strategy, the problem arises of how to demonstrate an impact of the intervention. Many ameliorative services find it quite easy to achieve visibility for their successful outcomes, especially when their clients are grouped in institutions; whereas it is much more difficult to show to policy makers or to the general public that children at-risk would have become disabled but for a given intervention. This difficulty of demonstration is all the more frustrating, since the number of clients who stand to benefit from the less visible, preventive strategies is always much greater than the number who can be accommodated in the institutional centres whose curative services attract so much publicity. As a result, a disproportionate amount of those scarce resources which have become available for rehabilitation services in TWCs have tended to be invested in conspicuous and relatively cost-ineffective institutions, or 'rehabilitation palaces' as Miles (1986) has dubbed them. The slow rate of acceptance of the more modest community-based approach advocated by the World Health Organization (WHO, 1980, 1983) has probably as much to do with impressionistic judgments by politicians as with resistance by quality-conscious professionals.

The designation of a child as at-risk for disability is based on the notion that a specific causal connection has been established between certain antecedent conditions and particular forms of disability. This has sometimes been held to include the correlation between certain socio-cultural and/or economic characteristics and average levels of achievement in a public school system. The interpretation of such correlations is however highly controversial (Jensen, 1969; Scarr, 1981; Cole and Bruner, 1971; Howard and Scott, 1981). In our view it would be very unwise in countries of the Third World to extend the criteria of risk to include membership of economically disadvantaged and/or culturally marginal groups. Rather we would suggest that risk be defined in individualized terms with reference to observable indicators of organic deficiency and/or delayed behavioural development, or specific hazards in the child's immediate and effective environment.

One of the most widely cited risk factors in TWCs is malnutrition. The most important long-term strategy for combatting this scourge is macro-economic planning to ensure improved levels of food production and distribution. While severe malnutrition can undoubtedly cause irreversible brain damage, the available evidence suggests that most children treated for mild or moderate levels of malnutrition will display only minor and temporary retardation of development. A secondary risk, however, is the 'behavioural vicious circle' of diminishing social interaction between mother and infant (Dasen and Super, 1988). A strategy for identifying individuals at special risk in this respect, within the context of the widely followed practice of growth-monitoring at health centres, may hold the prospect of preventing the occurrence of severe disabilities at the most vulnerable tail end of the distribution.

EPIDEMIOLOGY AND DETECTION

Technical Problems

Global estimates to the effect that 10% or more of the world's children are disabled, amounting to some 140 million disabled children of whom 120 million live in the Third World (Rehabilitation International, 1981) have a technically very tenuous foundation. Undoubtedly childhood disability occurs in all the countries of the world, and the population of the Third World is both larger and demographically younger than that of the more industrialized countries. But there is no reliable data base for estimating how many of the TWCs' millions of children have specifiable disabilities. Numerous scattered reports are available from various TWCs which provide details of aetiology and degrees of severity for samples of disabled clients seen at a referral centre. Such studies, however, do not afford an overall picture of the problem (Saunders, 1984). On the other hand, estimates based on the epidemiology of disability in industrialized countries where most of the general population surveys have been conducted are liable to provide a somewhat misleading account of the frequency of various types of condition likely to be encountered in TWCs.

Because of the scarcity of full-scale epidemiological studies of disability in TWCs, planners have been forced to speculate. One plausible hypothesis which has been frequently advanced is that, given the relatively poor obstetric and antenatal care prevailing in these countries, the incidence of conditions such as severe intellectual disability (mental retardation), is likely to be higher than the rates reported for countries such as Sweden, UK or USA with more highly developed maternal health services (Tizard, 1972; Belmont, 1981; Wiesinger, 1986).

An important distinction must be drawn, however, between incidence and prevalence rates. Incidence refers to the rate of occurrence in a given population of a particular disabling condition, while prevalence refers to the number of persons displaying the disability in question within the total population. The incidence of a certain disabling condition (e.g. brain damage) may be high, but if the majority of the affected children die within a few months then the prevalence of the condition will be relatively low. Since many disabling conditions also render infants highly vulnerable to potentially fatal infections and other secondary complications, the high infant mortality common in TWCs may tend to reduce significantly the current prevalence rate of childhood disabilities. The paradoxical possibility must also be acknowledged that future advances in the quality and coverage of general health services may give rise to an increase rather than a decrease in prevalence, by raising the survival chances of certain categories of congenitally vulnerable children. This possibility has been advanced as one of the reasons for encouraging TWC planners to begin to take stock of what at present seems to many of them a relatively marginal issue (Belmont, 1981).

While TWCs share as part of their defining characteristics many important consequences of a relatively weak economy, they also vary widely in demographic profile, ecological features, history and culture. As a result, both the origins and the consequences of early childhood disability may be quite different in one Third World country from those in another, and the immediate value of screening for any particular disorder will vary accordingly. Recognizing this diversity, Fryers (1986) has proposed a checklist of criteria for deciding in a given TWC whether screening for particular disabilities is likely to be effective. These include: the importance of a given condition in terms of the social and economic burden it places on the community, knowledge of the likely course of its development in the absence of any specific intervention, the current feasibility of ameliorating the condition which available resources, the design of screening procedures suitable for use by relatively untrained personnel in remote areas, the local validity and reliability of the test(s) available, and the safety and cultural acceptance of the screening procedure eventually adopted. An important aspect of Fryers' criteria for screening is the emphasis he places on the relationship between assessment of the disability and the design of an intervention programme — a topic we take up in the next section.

ASSESSMENT AS A GUIDE TO ACTION

Assessment in the context of childhood disability can be seen to serve three functions:

1. to detect problems and help identify those with special needs
2. to diagnose causes, and prescribe appropriate types of intervention
3. to monitor change and help evaluate the impact of intervention (Serpell, 1987).

Item 1 represents the screening function discussed above, and it is often described as a preliminary exercise completely independent of 2, the diagnostic/prescriptive function of assessment. But in TWCs which have only small numbers of highly trained professionals, the two stages may, in practice, often need to be collapsed into one. Individual programme plans (IPP) of remedial intervention in these countries are generally supervised, if at all, by paraprofessional or voluntary community-based workers most of whom have access to very limited training in the techniques of assessment. Professional personnel responsible for ascertainment therefore have a golden opportunity, which may not recur at a later stage, to map out the framework of an IPP for the child on the occasion of initial identification. When doing so, they would also do well to specify some criteria for 3, monitoring and evaluation, since this will generally be undertaken partly by those responsible for implementation and/or supervision of the IPP and partly by other professionals, none of whom will have guaranteed access to those who initiated the intervention process.

Detection and Identification

Interest in early intervention for disabled children is of relatively recent origin in TWCs. As a result it is still a rather experimental field. There has thus been a tendency to adopt Western methods of assessment which may not always be appropriate. The most widely used form of assessment, especially for intellectual disability, has been that based on a set of reference norms. Here performance of an individual is assigned a score relative to that of a standardization sample of a general population. In this way, for example, an individual may be classified as mentally retarded or intellectually disabled on the basis of intelligence quotients (IQ).

Intelligence tests have been a subject of great controversy. One of the arguments against their use has been that they tend to simplify the concept of intelligence by reducing it to a single dimension while presenting an image of rigorously quantified objective measurement. There has therefore been a shift of emphasis away from an exclusive reliance on IQ scores in determining the need for intervention, towards a broader range of measures covering not only cognitive development, but also the development of social, communication, self-help and motor skills.

In TWCs one of the most serious objections to the use of intelligence tests is that few of them have been properly adapted and standardized for the relevant population. To interpret an individual's score on such a test with reference to norms derived from samples which are culturally alien can be grossly misleading (Serpell, 1988). On the other hand, a certain element of 'norm-referenced assessment' is essential to the detection of those cases which are to be regarded as problems deserving further investigation. Norm-referenced assessments has a number of valuable applications outside IQ tests. One of these applications has been the use of Growth Charts as a key element of UNICEF's strategy of 'GOBI and FFF' (Grant, 1984). These charts are based on the principle of comparing a child's weight to the statistical distribution of weights of children at that age in a standardization sample (Morley and Woodland, 1979). For the purpose of detecting problems especially of a biological nature, it is necessary to establish a cut-off point in relation to the range of normal variation.

Diagnosis, Prescription and Monitoring

However, if assessment is to be used as a guide to action it is more important to compare an individual's present condition to what is normal for him or her than to compare the person to other individuals. If a child, for example, starts to walk independently or to talk, and later loses the ability to do so, this may be an important indicator of the occurrence of some organic impairment. Furthermore, in diagnosing the cause of such impairment it is usually helpful to compare the level of development of one function to that of others. Impairment of certain motor or sensory functions, for example, often serves as a pointer to localized neurological damage.

In assessing intellectual disability, several domains of psychological functioning are usually examined. These include: learning and understanding new tasks; language and communication; gross and fine motor skills; self-help/maintenance skills; and skills of social cooperation (Serpell *et al.*, 1988). The profile of an individual's relative strengths and weaknesses across these various domains provides a basis for setting prioritites in the design of an IPP. Assessment schemes such as the Portage Guide to Early Education checklist (Bluma *et al.*, 1976) spell out a sequence of behaviours in the order in which competence is normally attained in the course of a child's development. An IPP in such cases can be designed to focus on assisting the child to master 'the next step on the ladder' (Simon, 1981) of developmental progress. such 'profile-referenced assessment' can thus serve both a diagnostic purpose and a prescriptive one as a guide to intervention. The profile, in addition to identifying major weaknesses and needs, can also be used to identify strengths on which a training programme can be built. Such an assessment can be extended in scope to include the family, the home and the community. A caregiver may unknowingly maintain undesirable behaviour by the child. Such a person is also in a strategically powerful position to stimulate, shape and maintain desirable new behaviours and to cultivate new skills. In order to realize this potential in the context of an intervention programme, the caregiver's own needs and skills must be assessed. These can only be understood in the context of the dynamics of the family and community.

One decision of crucial importance in home based learning is whom to entrust with the responsibility of implementing specific intervention procedures. In Zambia, failure to identify an effective resource person within the child's immediate family setting was found to be a common weakness in IPPs designed on the basis of rapid preliminary assessment (Serpell and Nabuzoka, 1985). Research is currently under way in a number of TWCs to explore ways of assessing the potential of a child's regular effective home environment for the promotion and support of his or her healthy psychological development (Kagitcibasi, 1984; Nikapota, 1987; Serpell, 1987). One of the products of the Zambian study which is still being field tested is a 'Home Environment Potential Assessment' schedule, analogous to, but also different in significant respects from the HOME inventory developed by Caldwell and Bradley (1984) for use in the USA. One of the potential applications envisaged for such an instrument is the identification of key resource persons in the home environment of a child with, or at risk for, developmental disability, who are likely to be able and willing to take responsibility for ameliorative and/or preventive intervention activities.

Another major approach to assessment is to examine performance in relation to the intrinsic content of a given task. Such 'criterion-referenced assessment' is especially helpful for monitoring a child's progress towards the set goals and for evaluating the impact of a particular intervention. Task analysis of the skills selected as objectives of an instructional curriculum yields items for inclusion in the test. A child can, for example, be assessed as to how well he or she can walk or talk or wash him or herself in terms of the proportion of elements of the task he or she has mastered. Such an assessment is without reference to other aspects of the profile of abilities or to the age at which other children achieve a given level of competence on the task or skill. The skill being assessed therefore needs to have functional value within the ecological setting (Baine, 1986) relevant to the child's present or probable future life situation. Then only can intervention be meaningful.

Service Coordination

In most TWCs, early detection and intervention are not routinely undertaken under the auspices of any of the major existing rehabilitation services, partly because the staff of these services are already overstretched. The detection of disabilities is usually done in an uncoordinated manner. A young child may be ascertained as disabled during a routine visit to a hospital or health centre, or through casual contact with a specialist teacher or even by a herbalist or traditional birth attendant, but the full implications of such assessment may not be explained to the parents and only a little advice may be given. In such instances systematic remedial assistance of the child is often delayed until the child is of school age. Moreover even at that age, in a number of cases the child's family may have decided that the child will not benefit from any formal education and thus not bother to try to enrol him or her in school.

The tendency for intervention often to be delayed until school age is partly due to the very restricted scope of preschool education, which is still quite a recent phenomenon in many TWCs and mainly confined to the urban elite, especially in Africa. Thus even parents who appreciate the potential value of early systematic stimulation and training for their child may simply not have access to any such early intervention services.

Examples from Third World Countries

Several TWCs have, however, undertaken attempts to formalize procedures for assessment, referral and early intervention. Within Africa, Ghana established a National Assessment and Resource Centre in Accra in order to assess children for school placement as well as those referred by hospital and parents. The centre was also mandated to offer guidance and counselling to parents and classroom teachers to enable them to understand the children and help them in learning (Ghana Ministry of Education, 1974; Nabuzoka, 1986). In Kenya, the Ministry of Education, Science and Technology has established 23 Educational Assessment and Resource Centres since 1984, where more than 3,000 children had been identified by 1987. These centres also provide peripatetic services for schools which have integrated handicapped children (Kristensen and Wabuge, 1987). Zimbabwe provides another example of assessment and support to teachers and parents. The School Psychological Services at Zimbabwe's Ministry of Education and Culture operate several centres spread throughout the country to ensure coverage of all schools and a smooth referral system for remedial education.

In the Caribbean, Early Assessment and Stimulation Projects were started in Jamaica in 1975, in Barbados in 1980, in Curacao in 1977, and in Haiti in 1986 (Thorburn, 1986).

In Asia, the Philippines Foundation for the Rehabilitation of the Disabled, in conjunction with the Mental Feeding Programme of the Nutritional Centre of the Philippines and UNICEF in 1979 launched a project entitled 'Reaching the Unreached'. The project was aimed at the elaboration of simple indicators for early detection of impairments and low-cost intervention measures using local resources for children of the 0–6 age group (Wong and Tompar-Tiu, 1981). In Sri Lanka, Nikapota (1984, 1987) has described a pilot programme for integrating child mental health within the framework of regular primary health care services. In all of the examples cited above, assessment is being used as a guide to active intervention programmes. Among them, two somewhat contrasting strategies to early intervention efforts may be distinguished, one focussed around specialized centres, the other based more diffusely in the community.

SPECIALIZED CENTRES AND COMMUNITY-BASED SERVICE STRATEGIES

The first formal paradigm of special education for children with various types of disability was established in Europe where specialists administered 'hands-on' treatment to their clients in separate institutions (Pritchard, 1963). This principle of confining (re)habilitation activities within the walls of a specialized centre was extended to hospitals, residential special schools and sheltered workshops, and had become established as the prevailing international orthodox tradition by the middle of the 20th century.

Such institutions were, and indeed often still are, regarded as centres of excellence whose highly trained, professional staff were uniquely well qualified to offer a specialized form of service. As a result, the model was often exported with little or no adaptation to TWCs as a starting point for service provision, and to this day a large proportion of the few rehabilitation services in these countries are based in conspicuous institutions located in large cities.

Limitation of Specialized Services

However, the publication of several major studies showing that institutionalization has many negative consequences, especially for the psychological development of young children in orphanages, gave rise in the Western industrialized countries during the 1960s to a growing barrage of criticism of this approach. It is now widely agreed among researchers that individualized attention and consistent emotional support are crucial ingredients of the environment required for healthy psychological development, particularly in a child's early years (Bronfenbrenner, 1979). These environmental characteristics are generally much more readily provided to children in a small family setting than in a large institution. Consequently there has been a move towards a new pattern of service provision for children (and adults) with special needs, in which professional interventions are as far as possible delivered to the client within the context of her natural family, or failing that, a foster home. In several industrialized countries, an explicit policy of de-institutionalization has been adopted with a timetable for closing down the existing residential centres and redeploying their inmates and their personnel in various forms of community living.

While the consequences of this social movement have yet to be fully evaluated (Carr, 1985; Clarke and Clarke, 1985; Mittler and Serpell, 1985), a number of supplementary reasons for de-emphasizing specialized centres in the provision of services for the disabled in TWCs are already worth noting. They are generally capital-intensive projects, which depend for their effectiveness on advanced and highly specialized training, and on sophisticated equipment procured at high cost from abroad and difficult to maintain. Moreover, by isolating disabled children from the mainstream of society they run significant risks of establishing curricula which are inappropriate as a preparation for normal community life, hence promoting permanent dependency among their clients, and of perpetuating public attitudes of fear or pity rather than full acceptance (Serpell, 1986).

Given the limited resources which TWCs can generally mobilize for rehabilitation services, and the fact that many disabled persons are widely scattered across rural areas, a more sociologically appropriate and economically realistic strategy appears to be that of diffusing technical advice to the families into which disabled children are born through public information media and generic health, education and social welfare service personnel. This community-based approach to intervention, which has been advocated by the World Health Organization (WHO) in collaboration with other specialized agencies of the United Nations (ILO, UNESCO, UNICEF), has a guiding principle that, whenever possible, direct, 'hands-on' services should be provided by members of the child's family and neighbourhood, within the context of the child's local home community, with professionals playing a supportive, back-up role. Such an approach requires relatively less funding to get started, while it addresses the needs of the total client population. Its effective implementation would also lead to a reduction in the number of children who may otherwise require institutionalization in the future (Marfo and Kysela, 1983).

Home-based programming offers several other advantages. The opportunity for full family participation in a habilitation process builds on the moral and emotional commitment to the welfare of a disabled child that generally exists within the family into which she or he is born. Relevant skills, knowledge and attitudes are imparted to parents and other members of the disabled child's family as they become more involved in the child's progress, and this in turn leads to a growth of confidence among members of the child's social environment in their competence to manage and overcome problems and to guide the child's development and progress. In terms of ensuring that disabled children acquire appropriate skills and/or behaviours, problems of transfer or generalization of learned behaviour are greatly minimized since behaviour is learned in the child's normal setting and remains subject to continuing reinforcement by the parents and/or some other relative. Furthermore the child's social adjustment and self-esteem stand to benefit from the family's natural focus on him or her as a whole person rather than one whose needs are fragmented or compartmentalized by the requirements of professional specialization (Serpell, 1986).

Community Based Programmes

Several TWCs have attempted community-based programmes for early intervention. In Jamaica, for instance, an early stimulation project designed to develop a low cost model for early intervention recruited a team of community women, a number of whom were parents of disabled children themselves, to make weekly visits to the homes of disabled children. Here they would demonstrate step-by-step to the parents, the activities to be undertaken for their child's development, after which the parents themselves would carry out the training of their child (Thorburn, 1981).

In Mauritius, APEIM, a national organization of parents, has established with professional support, a parent volunteer training project whose purpose is to provide group and home training to parents and volunteers in how to apply low cost, simple intervention techniques with children under seven years of age who are 'at risk' or possess a permanent handicapping condition. The concept of 'parents helping parents' is being emphasized by the project in that parents of disabled children are trained to become the teacher and therapist of their own child and then to teach these techniques to other parents. The volunteers pay visits to families on alternate weeks to encourage follow-up of activities decided on at group meetings and also to talk to other members of the household (APEIM, in press).

Another example of a community-based service in a TWC, which includes young children as well as older clients, is Zimbabwe's rural home-based learning programme. The programme was launched in 1985 by the Zimcare Trust, an umbrella agency established to coordinate the activities of all non-governmental bodies concerned with intellectual disability in Zimbabwe, and is designed to suit parents and lay helpers with very limited formal education. Zimcare staff and family support workers, in consultation with regular caregivers, usually the mother or grandmother, draw up IPPs for each child enrolled in the programme. The family supporters are responsible for visiting the home regularly, in most cases weekly, to monitor progress and adapt the teaching activities as necessary. Each of the family supporters visits about 25 families. The Zimcare staff make six-weekly visits to review work done by the local personnel and to assess new clients (Mariga, in press).

Similar community-based services have been attempted in Botswana (Sebina and Kgosidintsi, 1981), Zambia (Nabuzoka, 1983) and the Philippines (Wong and Tompar-Tiu, 1981). In these programmes, the strategy has been to pass on skills from professionals to frontline workers who would in turn pass them on to the child's primary caregiver and/or other family members.

The community-based rehabilitation (CBR) approach has not escaped criticism. Miles (1986) in particular, has drawn attention to significant shortcomings in the WHO Manual, Training Disabled People in the Community (1980, 1983). It is arguable that the goals of CBR are unattainable given the limited training and experience available to families and grass-roots workers in most parts of the Third World combined with their many competing responsibilities. Moreover there may be a danger of 'selling short' the most needy disabled persons and families if hard-pressed policy-makers come to conceive of CBR as a cheap option for the rural poor. If CBR is to fulfill its promises of promoting full participation, normalization and acceptance, genuine technical support must be provided to those entrusted with 'hands-on' responsibilities, in the form of training, regular visiting and back-up (Serpell, 1986).

In a number of countries a middle way is being sought between community-based services and those provided by specialized centres. In Pakistan, for instance, community centres are being promoted to which disabled children come during the day (Miles, 1986). These centres are designed to aid a Community Rehabilitation Scheme while also aiming at achieving a higher level of professional competence. Thus personnel are trained through short orientation courses with a view to setting up other small centres elsewhere. The idea is to have a strong regional resource and training centre from which a number of small units would spring. The idea of resource centres for special education is also being promoted in other countries such as Kenya (Kristensen and Wabuge, 1987) and Ghana (Nabuzoka, 1986). One of the functions proposed for those centres is to serve as a base for peripatetic services which, by emphasizing mobility of specialist personnel, would alleviate the shortage of specialized manpower.

TRAINING NEEDS AND CURRICULA

Whether an early intervention programme is conceived as preparatory for centre-based or community-based rehabilitation services, it is clear that certain aspects of the work will call for special kinds of orientation and training. Much of the essential 'hands-on' work with very young children in a TWC will necessarily take place within their home environment. Families bring to such a task many strengths, but also stand to benefit from technical advice. A major challenge facing most TWCs is how to make its limited current resources of relevant specialized scientific knowledge and professional expertise as accessible and effective as possible for the majority of the children in need of them.

Thorburn and Roeher (1986) have underlined the importance of examining the total system within which service delivery is envisaged. Several levels of personnel can be identified, at each of which different amounts and types of training will be required. In the frontline are the trainers (WHO, 1983) or implementers (Wirtz, 1981) who are in continuous daily contact with the child: family members, volunteers and direct-care staff. Their needs are mainly for short, structured, 'on-the-job' courses of skill training, although their emotional needs for moral support and encouragement should also not be neglected (Sandow, 1984). The next level comprises local supervisors (WHO, 1983) or resource-persons (Nabuzoka, 1983), most of whom in TWCs are recruited from the ranks of primary health care workers, primary school teachers and community development personnel. TWCs which have attempted to mount early intervention programmes have generally preferred courses at this level also to be only of short duration, ranging from about two to eight weeks, since the trainees best placed to do the work can seldom be released for training for a longer period of time. On-the-job training with repeated cycles is sometimes ideal, since it provides built-in opportunities for demonstration and practice.

These two groups of people are often somewhat misleadingly called 'aides', as if their role were ancillary to the work of more senior, professional personnel. In practice, most of their work is autonomous and when they come into occasional contact with highly trained specialists, the latter rely on the former's local cultural knowledge and intuitions to guide the application of techniques to the unique situation of a particular client family (Climent, 1982; Serpell, 1982; Mittler and Serpell, 1985). These encounters are therefore more properly regarded as occasions for sharing skills than as supervisory checks by superiors on the work of subordinates. Werner and Bower (1982) and Werner (1987) provide a wealth of learning resources for promoting the resourcefulness expected of community-based workers in a TWC.

The third level of personnel comprises the cadre whose specialized training needs have been most widely recognized, such as physiotherapists, psychologists, specialist teachers of persons with visual, hearing, or intellectual disabilities, and orthopedic technicians. The ratio of personnel with these types of specialization to their target clientele in most TWCs is likely, in the foreseeable future, to remain inadequate for them to work directly with more than a tiny proportion of the children who could benefit from their skills. Thus there is a need to make the few available professionals aware of their obligation to pass on as much as possible of their 'know-how' to colleagues at the first two levels described above. Such a diffusion of skills seems to require rather a substantial reorientation of the pattern of training offered to these professionals. Their training should explicitly prepare them for the tasks of explaining to others the techniques they have acquired, teaching others to apply those techniques and evaluating how well these taught skills have been mastered. The community-based programmes cited earlier clearly exemplify this type of delegated expertise. In Zimbabwe, for example, a small team of professionals have trained, supervised and monitored the work of paraprofessionals in some rural areas who, in turn, demonstrate the skills to families with an intellectually disabled child for implementation

(Mariga, 1987). Clearly, communication skills and instructional methods should be included in the training curriculum for the professionals who are expected to lead or supervise such community based programmes.

A fourth level of personnel is required for central planning and management of services and for certain key roles in referral centres. Typically those roles are performed by senior professionals promoted from level 3. Much of the controversy over the releative merits of centre-based and community-based service strategies arises from the fact that earlier generations of specialists had little opportunity to conduct outreach work. As more specialists become aware of the importance of this dimension of service provision, its incorporation in medium-term planning will become easier. Planning involves an important element of advocacy, especially in TWCs where, as we noted above, considerable political resistance is often encountered. In-service seminars and conferences can serve a valuable function at this level by affording specialists, politicians and bureaucrats opportunities to confront one another's perspectives, to talk through their misconceptions and to identify common ground. International (especially regional and sub-regional) meetings can also serve as important catalysts by making TWC planners aware of what is feasible in countries which face similar economic problems to their own, and by generating concrete projects of cooperation.

APPROPRIATE TECHNOLOGY AND COMMUNICATION STRATEGIES

We have discussed in earlier sections why it is important in TWCs to rethink or adapt methods of assessment, service design and training developed in and for quite different societies in the industrialized world. The problems posed by this aspect of the transfer of technology are sometimes overlooked on the assumption that the necessary adaptation of imported industrial products to local purposes is a simple matter of common sense.

A useful distinction to emerge in the computer age is that between technological 'hardware' and 'software'. In principle a machine, a building or a gadget (hardware) imported from another society should be programmable (software) to serve the particular cultural, social, political and economic needs of the recipient. Motor cars, for instance, may be driven on whichever side of the road local decision-makers determine, and at whatever speed, over whatever terrain, and by whatever categories of driver. New regulations, training and minor hardware adaptations (such as special tyres, alternative fuels) may be required, but the versatility of the machine is such that an illusion of complete control is easily acquired by the importing society. The easiest constraint to detect is affordability; most TWCs have now have now become acutely conscious of their economic dependence on producer countries for the supply of spare parts (more hardware), and have responded by trying to localize production and maintenance capacity. But there are other, more insidious consequences of adopting a particular technological solution to one's problems. Reliance on motorized transport, for instance, has probably served to compound the stratification of TWC societies into a centralized rich, urban, industrialized sector and peripheral, poor, rural, 'underdeveloped', 'inaccessible' communities. The possibility of rapid travel, albeit only over selected parts of the country, and the resulting changes in administrative practices have tended to redefine the problems of service delivery in terms of 'accessibility'.

A somewhat analogous short-cut solution to the problems of psychological assessment is the adoption of Western IQ tests, which can easily result in anomalous definition of certain children as 'untestable', or of certain broad sections of a TWC society as intellectually 'backward' (Serpell, 1988). Likewise a superficial transfer of the concept of environmental enrichment has sometimes been used to justify the supply of largely irrelevant, imported toys and puzzles to rural communities in TWCs, rather than attempting to mobilize their indigenous cultural resources (Ivic, 1987).

Unpackaging and Adapting Technology

The implication we draw from this analysis is not that TWCs have nothing to learn from technological developments in the industrialized countries, but rather before borrowing from that technology it should be unpackaged (Cherns, 1984; Serpell, 1984). The basic theoretical rationale for a given artifact should be considered first for its relevance to an understanding of the recipient society's problem, and thereafter each factor contributing to the original design of the artifact should be carefully evaluated for its local applicability. A useful guide to this process in the case of an early intervention programme will be what Baine (1986) has called an 'ecological inventory', specifying the major demands imposed on a growing child by the local physical and cultural environment. Another key principle should be that of matching the operational and maintenance demands of any new technology to the skills and understanding of the recipient community.

Caston and others have developed impressive models of prosthetic and assistive devices for children with movement disabilities which can be constructed by local craftsmen or women in most TWC communities from locally available and affordable materials. Excellent illustrated publications of such designs for appropriate rehabilitation devices and techniques are available (at minimal cost to subscribers in TWCs) from AHRTAG (the Appropriate Health Resources and Technologies Acting Group, 85 Marylebone High Street, London W1M 3DE, UK). Other, somewhat more complex devices, such as wheelchairs, spectacles and hearing-aids can also be produced in TWCs by establishing low-cost industrial workshops at enormous savings relative to imported products, but these projects require some initial capital investment and political support to protect them from unfair competition.

Sharing Skills and Empowerment

Training also plays an essential role in ensuring an optimal level of decentralization. General surgeons based in community hospitals, for instance, can rapidly be taught the skills of club-foot surgery. Many eye and ear infections can be detected and treated by primary health care personnel with powerful consequences for the effective level of stimulation impinging on a young child. Another cadre of people whose potential role in early intervention has still to be fully recognized and promoted is the large network of traditional birth attendants and health practitioners whose practices are often intimately tied to prevailing parental beliefs (Peltzer and Kasonde-Ng'andu, 1987). For instance, in a number of TWC communities, tradition dictates that a newborn child be examined closely for detection of any possible defects, and that various types of manipulation and massage of the limbs be systematically taught to a young mother as part of the daily care for her infant.

One of the most widely applied software technologies for early intervention is behaviour modification. Although it is arguable that some of its potential has been under-realized due to 'cook book approaches' and 'oversimplification' (Kiernan, 1985), the dissemination of behaviourist principles has made a very considerable impact on special education in general but especially on home-based learning programmes. The concepts of task analysis, reinforcement, shaping, chaining and generalization are easily conveyed and have wide application. Much of the popularity of the Portage Guide to Early Education (Bluma *et al.*, 1976) in various TWCs (Jesien, 1983) may be attributed to its incorporation of these principles in a carefully elaborated, modular curriculum.

An important dimension of the home-based learning approach which we noted earlier is its focus on empowering the child's primary caregivers, building on and strengthening their moral and emotional commitment to the child's welfare, and capitalizing on their round-the-clock access to the child. In the domain of communication, Nwanze (1986, 1987) has recognized a powerful convergence of these ethical and practical considerations with the implications of contemporary 'pragmatic' theories of language development (Halliday, 1975; Bruner, 1975; Schieffelin and Ochs, 1986). Many researchers now agree that the inter-subjective understanding between mother and infant (Trevarthen, 1980) lays the essential foundations of communicative competence. If the intuitive knowledge of mothers in this domain can be mobilized and reinforced by professionals drawing their attention to the reciprocal relations between their own communicative behaviour and that of a child whose language development is delayed, the notion of parents as language therapists (Rees, 1982) may prove to have wide cross-cultural applicability (see Chapter Nine by Price and Bochner). Nwanze's exploratory research in

Nigeria suggests that mothers who were given such orientation with the aid of video-recordings modified their style of interaction with their children and that the latter's speech development improved accordingly.

A good example of a fully articulated programme for the detection and amelioration of childhood disabilities developed in and for a TWC is Zimcare's home-based learning programme. Specific assessment and instructional materials have been locally developed in each of the three major national languages of English, Shona and Ndebele, covering the topics of infant stimulation, self-help skills, language, motor skills, socialization, epilepsy and behaviour modification. Because the programme was designed to suit parents and lay helpers, a manual of teaching activities has been developed specially for use in rural communities. The manual, also in three languages, consists, following the Portage tradition, of a Teacher's Guide describing suitable activities related to performance levels on minimal tests, and a series of cards each specifying a set of activities illustrated with simple line drawings, which can be given to a client family (Mariga, 1987).

More recently this package has been supplemented with a series of videotapes, also locally produced, in which rural and urban Zimbabwean children with various types of disability are shown receiving specific types of stimulation and guidance in the context of their home communities (Mariga, McConkey and Mandiki, 1985). Although the hardware required for making and showing video is of foreign origin, the medium has proved to be highly adaptable to local conditions and requirements. By illustrating the interventions in a concrete manner, it is able to communicate effectively with people of limited formal education, and its durability and portability has made it possible to replicate richly illustrated courses for front-line and level 2 personnel in many parts of the country without placing unreasonable demands on the time of a very small, centrally-based professional team. The strategy appears to have wide applicability in TWCs (McConkey, 1986).

LOGISTICS OF PROGRAMMING AND EVALUATION

If the considerations outlined in papers and books like this one are to make a significant contribution to practice, their theoretical relevance must be translated into operational procedures. This is most easily achieved for a specific individual, more difficult to generalize to the design of a service project for a client population whose particular needs are not yet identified, and most difficult of all to build into a full-scale national or regional programme. By convention a new idea should be tested in practice within the framework of a pilot project of limited scope and duration before it is adopted as the basis for national, long-term policy; and none of the models of early intervention in TWCs can claim yet to have moved beyond this pilot phase.

'Going to scale', as Myers (1984) and others have pointed out, involves a broadening of objectives and a certain loss of focus by comparison with a pilot project. Large scale planning places greater emphasis on the inputs required, on hierarchical relations, on formal training and credentials; and the resulting bureaucracy can scarcely hope to retain the personal and flexible supervision often found within a successful pilot project. One strategy for countering these negative bureaucratic tendencies is deliberately to foster a diversity of local initiatives. Local groups of parents, linked and supported by a national 'umbrella', non-governmental organization, have proved in several European countries to be an effective means of maintaining accountability among service professionals towards their clients' families (Mittler and McConachie, 1983). Attempts to promote a similar model in Asian (Mittler and Beasley, 1982) and African (Serpell, 1982) countries are still at an early stage of development. It remains to be seen whether the relatively prosperous families which have taken an initiative in these TWCs will be able to represent the needs of the majority of client families.

A focus on early intervention is likely to appeal predominantly to professionals, since many parents (especially in countries with very scarce service provision) tend naturally to become preoccupied with the needs of older disabled children and adults, and an even greater preoccupation with the needs of adults tends to characterize self-advocacy movements of disabled persons. For this reason, and also for the sake of coordination and continuity of service provision, national professional organizations and governments have a crucial role to play in the planning of early intervention programmes in TWCs. Yet a number of constraints have been encountered in those TWCs where projects have sought to shift the emphasis of professional services towards the community-based approach advocated earlier (Thorburn, 1986). Generic service personnel are often overburdened with multiple tasks; some of them lack the positive attitudes towards disabled children required to motivate them to accept the additional responsibility of working with them; rigidity in the administrative system of these services also tends to inhibit such an expansion of their scope; and monitoring the quality of services provided by a widely scattered network of part-time personnel is logistically difficult for a small team of specialists.

Part of the problem seems to arise from the temptation to mount pilot projects on an artificially privileged scale which militates against the possibility of their widespread replication. Such projects are often conceived as some kind of blueprint or idealized model, and because their aspirations appear unrealistic to those working in the less privileged mainstream of service provision, no serious attempt is made to incorporate them in long-term national planning. Instead they remain the responsibility of a small group of enthusiasts relying on external financial support or, if that is withdrawn, gradually wither away. Korten (1980) has provided a powerful analysis of why some community-based development projects in TWCs in Asia have succeeded in gradually going to scale while many others have not. The key to their success, he suggests, lies in their adoption of a 'learning process approach', seeking to establish 'organizations with a well developed capacity for responsive and anticipatory adaptation – organizations that (a) embrace error; (b) plan with the people; and (c) link knowledge building with action' .

The recruitment, training and deployment of mobile specialists appears to be one of the key requirements for a wide-scale and effective early intervention programme in a TWC. In countries such as Zambia, with large, sparsely populated rural areas, reliable transportation becomes a high priority (Nabuzoka, 1983). Irrespective of population density, a large number of clients can be envisaged whose progress can only be monitored intermittently by a given specialist. This points to the need for an efficient record system to keep track of IPPs over quite long periods of time. Even in Britain where a generally high level of literacy prevails, Sandow (1984) reports that many parents evinced boredom or resentment towards the demand that they maintain detailed records of their disabled child's progress. In many TWCs this problem is likely to be compounded by low levels of functional literacy. Recording will thus become a major responsibility for the level 2 personnel in direct, regular contact with families. If they are to carry out this work precisely and conscientiously, they will need to appreciate its value. It should therefore receive special attention in their training, and regular opportunities should be provided for people working at this level to analyze and interpret the records they are required to generate (Serpell, 1982).

More generally, the processes of monitoring and evaluation, both for IPPs and for community programmes of early intervention are important opportunities for two-way communication, between service providers and clients, and between local and national (or sub-national) levels of programme management. Notions such as 'supervision' and 'quality control' need to be tempered with considerations of accountability. The political rhetoric of 'planning with the people' can only be translated into social reality if parents, families and communities are able to inject their felt needs into the formative evaluation of an unfolding programme.

CONCLUDING RECOMMENDATIONS FOR PRACTICE

1. Early intervention in TWCs should be focussed on the prevention or amelioration of disability in children with identified organic deficiencies and/or delayed behavioural development and in children whose immediate effective environment contains specific hazards.
2. Screening for this purpose should concentrate on conditions thought to place a significant burden on the community, unlikely to be self-correcting and for which amelioration is feasible with available resources.

3. Procedures used for screening should:
   a) be standardized for the local population,
   b) specify apparent trends over time in the individual's level of functioning,
   c) provide a profile of the individual's strengths and weaknesses across several domains,
   d) provide some preliminary guidance on how intervention should proceed.
4. Ideally the guidance for intervention provided by professional assessment should:
   a) provide a profile of the individual's needs and strengths,
   b) assess key features of the child's current effective home environment,
   c) identify strengths in the home on which an individualized programme plan (IPP) of amelioration can build,
   d) map out the framework of an IPP,
   e) specify criteria for monitoring the progress of its implementation, and
   f) specify criteria for evaluating its impact.
5. Early intervention should give priority to ensuring that the child's regular effective environment provides individualized attention and consistent emotional support. The most effective way of doing so in most TWCs will normally involve strengthening the family into which the child is born, or in exceptional cases, placement of the child in a small foster home.
6. Such home-based programmes should aim to build on the moral and emotional commitment of the family towards the child's welfare, by recruiting their fullest possible participation in the design and implementation of an IPP, by imparting new skills to them, thus further empowering them as effective habilitation, socialization and care providers, and by drawing their attention to the child's strengths, needs and progress.
7. Several levels of personnel are required for the effective implementation of community and home-based programmes of early intervention, and suitable training should be organized at each level.
   a) For front-line and community-level supervisory personnel, short on-the-job courses in repeated cycles will usually be most suitable.

b) Professional staff should be prepared explicitly for the tasks of explaining to others the rehabilitation techniques they have mastered, training others in those same skills and evaluating how well they have been learned.

c) Opportunities for multisectoral exchange of ideas should be provided to senior professional and administrative staff.

8. Equipment, techniques (such as tests and teaching methods) and programmes developed for early intervention work in industrialized countries should be carefully unpackaged and assessed before adoption for use in TWCs. Basic principles rather than concrete practices should form the starting point for evaluation and adaptation of imported technology to conform with the needs and resources of the recipient society.

9. New techniques which are considered locally applicable should be made available with appropriate training to as wide a spectrum of potential agents as possible, including parents, other family members, front-line personnel of generic education, health and social services and traditional health practitioners.

10. Behaviour modification, enhancement of mother-infant communication and video teaching represent three major technological strategies with widespread applicability for early intervention in TWCs.

11. Peripatetic mobility and intersectoral cooperation are key requirements for professional staff involved in early intervention programmes in TWCs.

12. Given the intermittent availability of such staff for monitoring individual clients' progress, techniques of accurate recording are an essential part of the training required by community level personnel entrusted with regular support of the front-line agents.

13. Client families and communities should be fully involved in the setting of targets for services and in the monitoring and evaluation of their attainment.

REFERENCES

APEIM (1987) 'The Parent Volunteer Training Project: An Early Intervention Model in Mauritius,' in R. Serpell, D. Nabuzoka and F. E. A. Lesi (eds), *Early Intervention to Prevent or Ameliorate Mental Handicap and Developmental Disabilities in Children of Pre-school Age in Africa* , (in press) Proceedings of a Sub-regional Workshop, June 1987, University of Zambia, CAMHADD, UNICEF, NORAD, Lusaka, Zambia,

Baine, D. (1986) 'Testing and Teaching Handicapped Children and Youth in Developing Countries,' UNESCO (*Guides for Special Education, No. 3*; ED-86/WS/59), Paris.

Belmont, L. (ed.) (1981) 'International Studies of Severe Mental Retardation,' *International Journal of Mental Health, 10*, (Special Issue).

Bluma, S., Shearer, J., Frohman, A., and Hilliard, J. (1976) *Portage Guide to Early Education*, CESA £12, Portage Wisconsin, USA (NFER/Nelson, Windsor, UK).

Bronfenbrenner, U. (1979) *The Ecology of Human Development*, Harvard University Press, Cambridge, Massachusetts.

Bruner, J. S. (1975) 'The Ontogenesis of Speech Acts,' *Journal of Child Language*, 2, 1–19.

Caldwell, B. M. and Bradley, R. H. (1984) *Home Observation for Measurement of the Environment*, (Rev. Ed.), University of Arkansas, Little Rock, Arkansas.

Carr, J. (1985) 'The Effect on the Family of a Severely Mentally Handicapped Child,' in A. M. Clarke, A. D. B. Clarke, and J. M. Berg (eds), *Mental Deficiency: The Changing Outlook* (4th ed.), Methuen, London, UK.

Cherns, A. (1984) 'Contribution of Social Psychology to the Nature and Function of Work and its Relevance to Societies of the Third World,' *International Journal of Psychology*, 19, 97–111.

Clarke, A. M. and Clarke, A. D. B. (1985) 'Life-span Development and Psychosocial Intervention,' in A. M. Clarke, A. D. B. Clarke and J. M. Berg (eds.), *Mental Deficiency: The Changing Outlook* (4th ed.), Methuen, London, UK.

Climent, C. E. (1982) 'Challenges in the Utilization of a Triaxial Classification of Disease in a Primary Health Care Setting,' in M. Lipkin and K. Kupka (eds), *Psychosocial Factors Affecting Health*, Praeger, New York.

Cole, M. and Bruner, J. S. (1971) 'Cultural Differences and Inferences about Psychological Processes,' *American Psychologist*, 26, 867–876.

Dasen, P. R. and Super, C. M. (1988) 'The Usefulness of a Cross-cultural Approach in Studies of Malnutrition and Psychological Development,' in P. R. Dasen, N. Sartorius and J. W. Berry (eds.), *Health Human Development: Applications from Cross-cultural Psychology*, Sage, California.

Fryers, T. (1986) 'Screening for Developmental Disabilities in Developing Countries: Problems and Perspectives,' in K. Marfo, S. Walker & B. Charles (eds), *Childhood Disability in Developing Countries: Issues in Habilitation and Special Education*, Praeger, New York.

Ghana Ministry of Education (1974) *New Structure and Content of Education for Ghana*, Ghana Publishing Corporation, Tema, Ghana.

Grant, J. P. (1984) *The State of the World's Children*, Oxford University Press, Oxford, UK.

Halliday, M.A.K. (1975) *Learning How to Mean: Explorations in the Development of Language*, Arnold, London, UK.

Howard, A. and Scott, R.A. (1981) 'The Study of Minority Groups in Complex Societies,' in R.L. Munroe, R.H. Munroe and B.B. Whiting (eds), *Handbook of Cross-Cultural Human Development*, Garlands STPM Press, New York.

Ivic, I. (ed.) (1987) *Traditional Children's Games*, OMEP, Belgrade, Yugoslavia.

Jensen, A. R. (1969) 'How Much Can We Boost IQ and Scholastic Achievement?,' *Harvard Educational Review, 39*, 1–123.

Jesien, G. (1983) 'Preschool Intervention Programs in Developing Countries: Why — and One Example of How,' *Portage Project, CESA* £12, Unpublished manuscript, Portage, Wisconsin.

Kagitcibasi, C. (1984) 'Socialization in Traditional Society: A Challenge to Psychology,' *International Journal of Psychology, 19*(1/2), 145–157.

Kiernan, C. (1985) 'Behaviour Modification,' in A. M. Clarke, A. D. B. Clarke and J. M. Berg (eds), *Mental Deficiency: The Changing Outlook* (4th ed.), Methuen, London, UK.

Kristensen, K. & Wabuge, R. (1987) 'Educational Assessment and Resource Services as a Strategy for Early Identification and Early Intervention of Children with Handicap,' in R. Serpell, D. Nabuzoka and F. E. A. Lesi (eds.), *Early Intervention to Prevent or Ameliorate Mental Handicap and Developmental Disabilities in Children of Pre-school Age in Africa*, (in press), Proceedings of a Sub-regional Workshop, June 1987, University of Zambia, CAMHADD, UNICEF, NORAD, Lusaka, Zambia.

Marfo, K. and Kysela, G. M. (1983) 'Rationale and Strategies for Early Intervention with Handicapped Children in a Developing Country,' in K. Marfo, S. Walker & B. Charles (eds), *Education and Rehabilitation of the Disabled in Africa, Vol. 1: Towards Improved Services*, Centre for International Education and Development, Edmonton, Alberta.

Mariga, L. (1987) 'Learning Needs of Parents and Lay Helpers in Rural Communities for Home-based Education of Pre-school Children with Mental Handicaps,' in R. Serpell, D. Nabuzoka & F. E. A. Lesi (eds.), *Early Intervention to Prevent or Ameliorate Mental Handicap and Developmental Disabilities in Children of Pre-school Age in Africa*, (in press), Proceedings of a Sub-regional Workshop, June 1987, University of Zambia, CAMHADD, UNICEF, NORAD, Lusaka, Zambia.

Mariga, L., McConkey, R., and Mandiki, L (1985), *Hope for the Child*, ZIMCARE Trust, Videotape, Harare, Zimbabwe.

McConkey, R. (1986) *Video Training in Developing Countries*, St Michael's House, Dublin, Ireland.

Miles, M. (1984) *Where There is No Rehab Plan*, Mental Health Centre, Peshawar, NWFP, Pakistan.

Miles, M. (1986) 'Misplanning for Disabilities in Asia,' in K. Marfo, S. Walker and B. Charles (eds), *Childhood Disability in Developing Countries: Issues in Habilitation and Special Education*, Praeger, New York.

Mittler, P. and Beasley, D. (1982) *A Multi-national Family Training Workshop*, Report to UN and UNESCO, ILSMH, Brussels, Belgium.

Mittler, P. and McConachie, H. (eds) (1983) *Parents, Professionals and Mentally Handicapped People: Approaches to Partnership*, Croom Helm, London, UK.

Mittler, P. and Serpell, R. (1985) 'Services: An International Perspective,' in A. M. Clarke, A. D. B. Clarke & J. M. Berg (eds), *Mental Deficiency: The Changing Outlook* (4th ed.), Methuen, London, UK.

Morley, D. and Woodland, M. (1979) *See How They Grow*, Macmillan, London, UK.

Myers, R. G. (1984) 'Going to Scale,' *Paper presented at the Second Inter-agency Meeting on Community-based Child Development*, September, UNICEF, New York.

Nabuzoka, D. (1983) 'Childhood Disability in Zambia: A Report of the Pilot Follow-up Project for Disabled Children in Katete District,' *University of Zambia, Institute for African Studies* (mimeo), Lusaka, Zambia.

Nabuzoka, D. (1986) 'Special Education in Ghana: A Report of a Study Tour for Special Education Research at the University of Cape Coast,' *University of Zambia/Association of Commonwealth Universities (mimeo)*, Lusaka, Zambia.

Nikapota, A. D. (1984) 'Contribution of Integrated Mental Health Services to Child Mental Health,' *International Journal of Mental Health*, 12(3), 77–95.

Nikapota, A. (1987) 'Strengthening Community Participation,' *Paper presented at the International Conference on 'Promoting the Mental Health of Children and Youth'*, October, Ottawa, Canada.

Nwanze, H. (1986) 'Characteristics of Maternal Language to Language Competent and Language Delayed Children,' *Paper presented at the 20th International Congress of the International Association of Logopedics and Phoniatrics*, August, Toyko, Japan.

Nwanze, H. (1987) 'Modification of Parent-child Interaction Patterns for Language Remediation', *Paper presented at the International Congress of the International League of Societies for Persons with Mental Handicap*, August, Rio de Janeiro, Brazil.

Peltzer, K. and Kasonde-Ng'Andu, S. M. (1987) 'The Role of Traditional Healers Towards Children's Mental Handicap and Developmental Disabilities in Lusaka', in R. Serpell, D. Nabuzoka and F. E. A. Lesi (eds), *Early Intervention to Prevent or Ameliorate Mental Handicap and Developmental Disabilities in Children of Pre-school Age in Africa*, (in press), Proceedings of a Sub-regional Workshop, June 1987, University of Zambia, CAMHADD, UNICEF, NORAD, Lusaka, Zambia.

Pritchard, D. G. (1963) *Education of the Handicapped 1760–1960*, Routledge and Kegan Paul, London, UK.

Rees, R. J. (1982) *Parents as Language Therapists: A Study in Parent-professional Cooperation*, South Australian College of Advanced Education, Australia.

Rehabilitation International (1981) 'Childhood Disability: Its Prevention and Rehabilitation', *Assignment Children*, 53/54, 43–75.

Sandow, S. (1984) 'The Portage Project: Ten Years On', in T. Dessent (ed.), *What is Important About Portage?*, NFER/Nelson, Windsor, UK.

Saunders, C. A. (1984) 'Handicapped Children: An Epidemiological Study in Plateau State', in H. V. Curran (ed.), *Nigerian Children: Developmental Perspectives*, Routledge and Kegan Paul, London.

Scarr, S. (1981) *Race, Social, Class and Individual Differences in IQ*, Lawrence Erlbaum, Hillsdale, NJ.

Schieffelin, B. B. and Ochs, E. (eds) (1986) *Language Socialization Across Cultures*, Cambridge University Press, Cambridge, UK.

Sebina, D. B. and Kgosidintsi, A. D. (1981) 'Disability Prevention and Rehabilitation in Botswana', *Assignment Children*, 53/54, 135–152.

Serpell, R. (1982) 'Social and Psychological Constructs in Health Records: The Need for Adaptation to Different Sociocultural Environments', in M. Lipkin and K. Kupka (eds), *Psychosocial Factors Affecting Health*, Praeger, New York.

Serpell, R. (1984) 'Commentary: The Impact of Psychology on Third World Development', *International Journal of Psychology, 19*, 179–192.

Serpell, R. (1986) 'Specialised Centres and the Local Home Community: Children with Disabilities Need Them Both', *International Journal of Special Education, 1*(2), 107–127.

Serpell, R. (1987) 'The Potential of Home Environments for Promoting Healthy Psychological Development in Early Childhood: In Search of Indicators', *Paper presented at the International Conference on 'Promoting the Mental Health of Children and Youth'*, October, Ottawa, Canada.

Serpell, R. (1988) 'Childhood Disability in Sociocultural Context: Assessment and Information Needs for Effective Services', in P. R. Dasen, N. Sartorius and J. W. Berry (eds), *Health Human Development: Applications from Cross-cultural Psychology*, Sage, California.

Serpell, R. (1987) 'Psychological Assessment as a Guide to Early Intervention: Reflections on the Zambian Context of Intellectual Disability', in R. Serpell, D. Nabuzoka and F. E. A. Lesi (eds), *Early Intervention to Prevent or Ameliorate Mental Handicap and Developmental Disabilities in Children of Pre-school Age in Africa*, (in press), Proceedings of a Sub-regional Workshop, June 1987, University of Zambia, CAMHADD, UNICEF, NORAD, Lusaka, Zambia.

Serpell, R. and Nabuzoka, D. (1985) 'Community-based Rehabilitation for Disabled Children in Vulamkoko Ward: A Follow-up Study', *Paper presented at Workshop on IPSCD at IASSMD Congress*, April, New Delhi, India.

Serpell, R., Zaman, S. S., Huq, S., Ferial, S., Silveira, M. L. M., Dias, A. M. C. de S., de Campos, A. L. R., Narayanan, H. S., Rao, P. M., Thorburn, M. J., Halim, A. J., Shrestha, D. M., Hasan, Z. M., Tareen, K. I., Qureshi, A. A., and Nikapota, A. D. (1988) 'Assessment Criteria for Severe Intellectual Disability (Mental Retardation) in Various Cultural Settings', *International Journal of Behavioural Development, 11*(1).

Simon, G. B. (1981) *The Next Step on the Ladder, British Institute of Mental Handicap,* Kidderminster, UK.

Thorburn, M. J. (1981) 'Community Aides for Disabled Preschool Children in Jamaica', *Assignment Children, 53/54,* 117–134.

Thorburn, M. J. (1986) 'Early Intervention for Disabled Children in the Caribbean', in K. Marfo, S. Walker and B. Charles (eds), *Childhood Disability in Developing Countries: Issues in Habilitation and Special Education,* Praeger, New York.

Thorburn, M. J. and Roeher, G. A. (1986) 'A Realistic Approach to the Preparation of Personnel for Rehabilitation Services in Developing Countries', in K. Marfo, S. Walker and B. Charles (eds), *Childhood Disability in Developing Countries: Issues in Habilitation and Special Education,* Praeger, New York.

Tizard, J. (1972) *Epidemiology of Mental Retardation: Implications for Research on Malnutrition,* Symposia of the Swedish Nutritional Foundation XII.

Trevarthen, C. (1980) 'The Foundations of Intersubjectivity: Development of Interpersonal and Cooperative Understanding in Infants', in D. R. Olson (ed.), *The Social Foundations of Language and Thought: Essays in Honour of Jerome S. Bruner,* Norton, New York.

Werner, D. (1987) *Disabled Village Children,* Hesperian Foundation, Palo Alto, California.

Werner, D. and Bower, B. (1982) *Helping Health Workers Learn,* Hesperian Foundation, Palo Alto, California.

WHO (1980, 1983) *Training Disabled People in the Community: A Manual on Community-based Rehabilitation for Developing Countries,* World Health Organisation, Geneva, Switzerland.

Wiesinger, R. (1986) 'Disabled Persons in the Third World: Present Situation and Changing Prospects for the Future', *International Journal of Special Education, 1*(1), 21–34.

Wirtz, S. (1981) 'The Pragmatics of Language and the Mentally Handicapped: The Speech Therapist's Role', in W. T. Fraser and R. Grieve (eds), *Communicating with Normal and Retarded Children,* John Wright, Bristol, UK.

Wong, W. and Tompar-Tiu, A. P. (1981) 'A Community Programme in the Philippines: The Project Reaching the Unreached', *Assignment Children, 53/54,* 165–183.

FOOTNOTES

1. Authors' addresses:
   Dr. Robert Serpell, Associate Professor, Department of Psychology, University of Maryland, Baltimore County Campus, 5401 Wilkens Avenue, Baltimore, MD   21228.
   Mr. Dabie Nabuzoka, Research Fellow, Community and Occupational Health Research Programme, Institute for African Studies, University of Zambia, PO Box 30900, Lusaka, Zambia
2. We follow the terminological recommendations of Mittler and Serpell (1985) in preferring the expression 'intellectual disability' to others such as 'mental retardation', 'mental handicap', etc.
3. Excellent illustrated publications of such designs for appropriate rehabilitation devices and techniques are available (at minimal cost to subscribers in TWCs) from AHRTAG Resources, the Appropriate Health and Technologies Action Group, 85 Marylebone High Street, London W1M 3DE, UK.

6 ASSESSMENT FOR EARLY INTERVENTION; EVALUATING CHILD DEVELOPMENT AND LEARNING IN CONTEXT

Keith D. Ballard

INTRODUCTION

Assessment is a process in which various strategies are used to evaluate child learning and development, including evaluation of the cultural, social and physical contexts within which learning and development occurs. It would seem self-evident that early intervention for infants who have disabilities should begin with assessment of the child's developmental status and continue with ongoing evaluation of environmental support and programme effectiveness.

Yet, until recently, assessment has predominantly involved psychometric tests that provide data on a limited range of behaviours in a few constrained settings. Such an approach to assessment reflects medical diagnostic procedures, which attempt to classify various signs and symptoms into aetiological and prognostic categories (Johnson, 1982; Wallace and Larsen, 1978). The labelling that emerges from such testing is not especially useful for designing teaching programmes, and may even inhibit intervention efforts for some children when a prediction based on normative data is not optimistic about future learning.

Increasingly, however, the assessment literature has begun to address the complexity of human learning and the plasticity of development. In particular, recognition has emerged for the significance of the environment and behaviour–environment interactions for learning (Kendall, Lerner and Craighead, 1984; Voeltz and Evans, 1983). Such thinking has focused on ecological concepts and on the need to understand and assess contextual influences on children.

Bronfenbrenner (1979) conceived of the ecological environment as extending far beyond the immediate situation directly affecting the developing person and stressed the significance of linkages between settings such as the home, community and the broader social–political contexts within which the family functions. These ideas may at first seem somewhat abstract and removed from the immediate concerns of the practitioner who must generate data and suggest directions for a specific infant who has disabilities.

However, both assessment processes and assessment data should be viewed in context. This context includes such issues as the cultural–political system that may impact on the infant's present status and future life chances. For example, there seems a common pattern for indigenous people who are also ethnic minorities in their country to show higher infant mortality rates and lower educational and employment achievements than in the dominant culture in that country.

It also includes the particular professional, such as a psychologist and the type of data he or she collects. The developmental, social and educational models that professionals work from will be reflected in the way in which the infant is assessed and described and in the intervention strategies that are proposed from the assessment.

The present chapter indicates the implications of such an ecological perspective on assessment. The emphasis will not be on a detailed description of specific assessment devices, their uses and limitations. Such information is available in other sources (e.g. Fewell, 1984; Johnson, 1982; Sheehan, 1982). Rather, the present chapter focuses on identifying the questions that assessment might ask and the assumptions and implications of both the questions asked and the strategies used to answer those questions.

THE GOALS OF ASSESSMENT

An overriding factor that will help determine both the assessment strategies that are used, and the type of outcome data obtained involves the goals that the psychologist has for the assessment. The assessment may be aimed at a description of the infant's behaviour and general developmental status. Such a description may be the first part of a classification process that will aissign the child to a category of disability. This, in turn, may be a step toward accessing an appropriate intervention programme and related resources for the child and family.

A critical question involves the purpose of the assessment. Yet an answer to the question, 'Assessment for what?' is not easily arrived at. The goals set by each psychologist reflect the context within which that person works. A major part of that context involves the professional's personal perspectives on such issues as the limits or plasticity of child development, on the commonalities of experience or the uniqueness of children who have disabilities and of their families, and the psychologist's views on the ways in which the education system and community should meet the special needs of children and their families.

Psychologists are involved in all of these issues as they plan and carry out their assessments. They need to be aware that certain kinds of assessment data imply a certain model of assessment that will influence their conceptualization of the infant and his or her needs. Normative data, for example, derive from a statistical model in which points on a continuum are arbitrarily identified as discriminating 'normal' from 'abnormal' development, with related predictions for future achievements. Another example of possibly hidden assumptions influencing assessment involves the psychologists who work with the concept of 'least restrictive environment' (Vincent *et al,*, 1980) in planning early intervention and preschool services for children. Their assessment and subsequent placements will differ in significant ways from the data and planning that would be generated by psychologists who work with the concept of the 'non-restrictive environment' as the basis of community integration for families with infants who have special needs (Taylor *et al.*, 1986). In the former case, children will be categorized and they and their families may make early contact with segregated facilities providing special programmes. In the latter case, categorical labels are not part of assessment and resources would be located in a way that would support all children and families in regular preschool and community settings (Ballard, 1988).

The outcomes for children and families in the preceding example could differ radically, and the effects of assessment and subsequent intervention strategies may extend across many years. Such possibilities suggest that the psychologist and the assessment strategies that she or he uses may become influential components of family systems, helping determine their perceptions of their needs and rights and how they manage the disability.

Assessment, therefore, is not simply an issue of measurement and of recommending a next step. The assessment process itself should be seen as potentially reactive, with the person undertaking the assessment becoming a part of the many factors impacting on the family, and therefore on the child. In this respect alone, assessment is a complex process that demands a high level of expertise in the areas of evaluation and in understanding the contexts within which child learning and development occur.

It is important, therefore, to evaluate the various processes that may be used in assessment and the attempt to anticipate possible 'collateral outcomes' from these processes. Collateral outcomes are effects that were not intended as part of an action, but that may be more significant than the intended outcome itself. Collateral effects may be negative, such as the low expectation for learning that may result from a low score on a developmental scale, or positive, such as the community acceptance and understanding that may result from enrollment of infants who have disabilities in regular childcare or preschool facilities. In the following sections an attempt will be made to suggest potential collateral outcomes to which the assessing psychologist should be alert.

ASSESSMENT AND TESTING

Normative testing has traditionally been a dominant model across most areas of assessment and the field of infancy and early childhood has been no exception.

The most commonly used standardized techniques for assessment during infancy involve the tests developed by Gesell 1940; Gesell and Amatruda, 1947), Cattell (1940) and Bayley (1969). Gesell's intention was to assess developmental status in terms of the 'totality of an infant's effective functioning ... composed of motor, adaptive, personal–social and language behaviours...', all of which derived from what was assumed to be a 'maturational unfolding process generally unaffected by external influences' (Yang and Bell, 1975). Cattell (1940) intended to measure infant intelligence and saw her test as a downward extension of the Stanford-Binet. The Bayley test is presented as a Mental Scale, Motor Scale and the Infant Behaviour Record. The test is intended to establish a child's current developmental status in relation to others of similar age and the author does not recommend predicting a child's later abilities from the scale scores. Nevertheless, the usual inference from normative testing is that performance that deviates from the norm indicates pathology, while this finding in turn is usually seen as suggesting that future problems may derive from current developmental abnormalities. Identification of difference, therefore, is usually taken as a signal for intervention.

Yang and Bell (1975) suggest that all three of these traditional scales support a view that infant development and intelligence are 'relatively unencumbered by environmental influence' and involve a 'maturationally and genotypically controlled conception of development' (p. 175). All three tests 'have proven to be systematically poor predictors of later performance' (Yang and Bell, 1975, see also Dunst andRheingrover, 1982).

Assessment could leave aside the issue of prediction and simply evaluate current developmental status, but there are still significant issues demanding extreme caution in interpreting data from normative testing. Simeonsson, Huntington and Parse (1980), for example, suggest that while developmental scales may appear to be similar in content and purpose they may not give comparable results. They note that the Bayley Scales and the Griffiths (1970) test of infant abilities have been shown to give substantially different results in a study with 50 high-risk infants (Ramsay and Fitzhardinge, 1977) and that a study comparing the Bayley Scales with the Gesell Developmental Schedules using a sample of 21 infants with Down's syndrome (Eippert and Azen, 1978) showed that the tests did not yield the same developmental patterns and could not, therefore, be considered interchangeable. The normative model presents further problems for interpreting data when there is evidence that the individual being assessed may not be like the individuals who made up the normative sample. The

Bayley Scale, for example, compares each infant to others of his or her age in the standardization sample, a sample that includes only 'normal' children living at home and excludes 'prematures, institutional infants and those from bilingual homes' (Collard, 1972, p. 728). Given that the experiences and development of infants who have disabilities are unlikely to be 'normal', there are obvious difficulties in rationalizing the comparison of their performance with that of non-disabled children. Further problems emerge when assessment involves modifying the presentation of the test to the needs of the child's disability. When an examiner changes the guidelines for administering a test or test item, or changes response requirements, then test validity is clearly violated (DuBose, 1982). Also, there is evidence that, compared with non-disabled peers, preschool children who have disabilities show test scores that are more seriously depressed when they have been tested by an examiner not known to them (Fuchs *et al.*, 1985). Fuchs and his colleagues showed that tests are not simply a sample of responses to standard stimuli, but represent social interactions to which disabled and nondisabled children attribute different meanings. It would seem that, rather than being 'objective' tests, these assessments are 'subjectivized' by children who have disabilities in terms of their unique experiential backgrounds.

Given that infant learning and development is an interactive, reciprocal, social process (Kendall, Lerner and Craighead, 1984), then a single, normative comparison within limited performance and environmental constraints offers little information of value to early intervention. Nevertheless, such testing is still seen by some practitioners (e.g. Sailor and Guess, 1983, p. 232) as a first identifying step. Test users should know that when used outside the normative comparison group for that instrument then their data are not valid. They should also to be aware that such testing often carries a powerful impression of a 'scientific' model of assessment so that test results may be taken much more seriously than the validity and quality of the data warrants. A negative collateral outcome of such testing is that it reinforces inappropriate assumptions, practices and concepts such as categorization and labelling, well illustrated by the 'prominent physician' cited by Stratford (1985), who claimed he had not seen 'one mongoloid that has an educable IQ' (p. 149).

While prediction based on intelligence quotients and developmental quotients presents more unsolvable problems than useful information, the general issue of identifying infants at risk remains a major concern for research and practice. Various screening strategies will be briefly reviewed before alternatives to normative testing are examined.

SCREENING FOR DEVELOPMENTAL DISABILITIES

The difficulty of predicting later development is frequently noted in discussions on strategies for identifying infants at or near birth who may be at risk of handicapping conditions. Gentry and Adams (1978), for example, review research on three assessment areas of: medical examination; environmental, maternal and infant risk factors; and standardized tests (e.g. Denver Developmental Screening Test, Frankeburg, Dobbs and Fandal, 1967). Gentry and Adams (1978) note that while risk factors and screening test scores identify a relatively large proportion of infants who have severe disabilities, research shows that screening tests are only tentative indicators of developmental problems for most other infants.

Screening tests have been devised to provide a relatively quick and inexpensive identification of infants who may need further assessment. As Fewell (1983a) notes, however, it is important to be aware of the theoretical perspective that each instrument reflects. The Denver Developmental Screening Test, for example, was based on items from the Gesell Developmental Schedules and so reflects a maturational developmental perspective. Other reviews (e.g. Sheehan, 1982) of behaviour checklists used with infants show that many lack reliability and validity information and rely on norms derived from other tests and checklists. Such strategies, therefore, must be recognized as inappropriate for children from different cultures or different developmental experiences to the children in the normative group; as reflecting a maturational rather than transactional (interactive) model of development; and as providing data that may be overvalued because they have the spurious 'scientific validity' that publication sometimes seems to confer on tests.

THE ASSESSMENT OF INFANT COGNITION

Practitioners working from a developmental testing perspective have had only limited success with their attempts at global evaluations of infant development and intelligence. Psychologists interested in human cognition have developed alternative approaches which attempt to access infant cognitive skills. Two important contributions are noted, first that of the Piagetian cognitive approach and second Zelazo's information processing model

The Cognitive Perspective

Assessment strategies derived from a cognitive perspective have focused on specific concepts (e.g. object permanence, conservation) rather than general abilities that reflect age-related maturation and learning. The ordinal scales developed by Uzgiris and Hunt (1975) were designed to assess an infant's current functional level within the sensori–motor period of intellectual development (two weeks to two years of age). These scales are based on Piaget's theories which stress a uniform sequence of development through successive stages. The interpretation of such scales need not rely on norms because a concern with age-related levels is secondary to a qualitative description of the child's characteristic behaviour

Anastasi (1976) suggests that ordinal scales are similar to criterion-referenced tests in providing information on what the child is actually able to do. Information from such testing is often seen as more relevant for intervention than the data derived from normative comparisons. From this perspective, it might seem that tests such as the Uzgiris and Hunt scales should indicate what it is that the child should learn next in the theoretical sequence toward intellectual competence. Yet the theoretical notion that sensori–motor intelligence is reflected through gross and fine motor actions in infants and young children has been challenged by Zelazo (1982). This researcher argues that motor actions need not be a reflection of cognitive attainments or of central nervous system integrity, and that impaired motor skills in infants who have disabilities would make the interpretation of testing on the Uzgiris and Hunt scales of questionable validity. Zelazo supports his case from research on infant memory which shows that learning does occur independently of gross and fine motor performance in the sensori–motor period. From this perspective, Zelazo suggests than an information processing approach may be a valuable alternative assessment strategy that could indicate intact or impaired information processing ability within the first three years of life.

An Information Processing Perspective

Zelazo's perceptual-cognitive assessment procedures involve establishing infant expectancy by presenting and repeating an event (a toy car rolls down a slope and knocks over an object) and then introducing a 'moderately discrepant variation of the standard' (the object does not fall over when the car runs into it - Zelazo, 1982, p. 110). Observational and heart rate measures indicate the child's anticipation of the discrepant event. If the child shows such anticipation then it is inferred that 'elicited behaviours reflect the matching of an external event to an internal representation of that event' (p. 116).

Zelazo's research is a creative response to his criticism of infant tests such as the Bayley and the Uzgiris and Hunt scales which emphasize motor items and imitation of motor performances. Zelazo argues that while intact neuromotor functioning may validly imply intact intellectual ability, 'the problem is that a poor neuromotor performance need not announce impaired intellectual ability' (Zelazo, 1982 p. 108). Zelazo also suggests that children who have language delays or behaviour difficulties that limit their compliance with testing are at risk of being labelled as having lowered intellectual functioning through an inappropriate comparison with a nonhandicapped normative group. Such labelling may result in lowered parental and teacher expectations and so contribute to the origins of 'iatrogenic retardation' (Zelazo, 1982 p. 109).

Zelazo's assessment strategies might show that an infant with physical or communication handicaps is, nevertheless, achieving normal cognitive development at the time of assessment. Such a finding may have implications for the design of an early intervention programme. On the other hand, where a 'delay' in central processing ability is indicated by these testing procedures, there may still be an unwarranted negative outcome in terms of a poor prognosis for future development and related lowered expectations by those responsible for planning an intervention programme.

PROBLEMS IN TESTING INFANTS

The work of Zelazo addresses directly some of the problems of assessment of infants who have disabilities. Whereas tests such as the Bayley scales and Piagetian based scales were designed around the development and skill capabilities of infants without disabilities, Zelazo takes into account the fact that infants and young children who have disabilities cannot be thought of as if they had the same developmental experiences and response capabilities as their non-handicapped peers.

Nevertheless, Zelazo's work retains some of the problems associated with the testing strategies reviewed in the present chapter. Essentially, all of these tests focus assessment on the child. A focus on the child may reflect various developmental theories but does not clearly address human learning and development from a transactional perspective. For example, predicting future development or intelligence from a normative model requires the assumption of 'approximately equal opportunity for learning' (Hunt, 1974, p. 127), an assumption that cannot be supported from research on families, from research on the development of infants who have disabilities, or from a perspective of common sense.

It is difficult, therefore, to see what value there is in normative, static, 'psychometric snapshots' (Messick, 1983). It is not so difficult to suggest that a collateral outcome of such assessments may involve identification of developmental and learning problems as primarily existing within the child. Simply labelling the organism as abnormal or as damaged or as having a limited capacity for learning seems unlikely to encourage detailed examination of contextual environmental issues or even to motivate the planning and implementation of intervention programmes.

As an assessment strategy, infant testing represents measurement based on a very few responses obtained in a specific (usually constrained) setting. Such data may be of some value if the user does not intend to predict beyond the test setting. In assessment, however, it is almost certain that test data, often obtained in one session with the child, will be used as the basis for making inferences about the child's likely performance in other settings at other times. Given what is known about the significance of the environment and setting events for child behaviour (e.g. Kendall, Lerner and Craighead, 1984), making such inferences from test performance can no longer be justified.

BEHAVIOURS CHECKLISTS AS AN ASSESSMENT STRATEGY

Observation checklists of infant and young children's behaviour have increasingly become a part of 'assessment battery' type evaluations and of behavioural assessment. In principle, assessing a child against a list of behaviours and skills usually acquired within certain chronological time-frames could indicate both the child's achievements and deficits. Also, such an assessment would appear to have direct implications for intervention, identifying skills and understandings that need to be taught to 'fill in' or 'catch up' with normal developmental achievements. However, many of the problems that apply to standardized testing apply equally to checklist measures, with the result that there are similar difficulties in translating the assessment data into intervention goals and practice.

Sailor and Guess (1983), for example, note that checklist assessments like the Adaptive Behavior Scales have been used extensively as the basis for instructional objectives. These authors suggest that such assessment systems, available to teachers of children who have severe disabilities, fail because they do not contain relevant, functional and therefore teachable items, and they do not provide sequences of items that translate into meaningful long-term goals (p. 117). The main reasons that these checklist assessments are of such limited value for instructional design is seen by Sailor and Guess as arising from the fact that they are constructed without a knowledge of how the development of children who have disabilities differs from patterns of normal development upon which most standardized assessment systems are based. A further problem is that these assessment systems are presented as if skills are developed in isolation, when in fact skills are usually interrelated and reflect the demands of different environments. Sailor and Guess record an experience that will be familiar to many practitioners. This involved making visits to a classroom for children who have severe disabilities, with a lengthy period between each visit, and noting that the pupils were working on the same tasks each time with no discernible gains in performance.

The tasks are usually the preschool type items represented in assessment checklists, and it is increasingly recognized that programmes based on such a developmental approach frequently involve tasks that are neither age appropriate nor functional for children who have disabilities (Guess and Noonan, 1982).

Sailor and Guess propose that a more appropriate strategy is 'to generate a curriculum for each student that is relevant, functional and unique to the individual needs of that student' (p. 117). This is achieved by establishing educational goals and short-term objectives with a task analysis for achieving sequential steps toward that goal. Assessment in such a model involves systematic behavioural observations to establish basal levels and to evaluate current performance levels within the teaching programme.

Although Sailor and Guess do not see standardized assessment instruments as a useful source of instructional objectives, they do see them as a useful source of assessment ideas. Similarly, Voeltz and Evans (1983), while rejecting the 'test-train' approach associated with developmental checklists see some value in using checklists as general benchmark measures that allow programme assessment over time.

An assessment which suggests that the next item in the checklist sequence should be the teaching goal is not well founded in theory or practical experience. Such an assessment is essentially out of context. It is out of context in developmental terms because there is insufficient research on the development of children who have disabilities on which to base assessments. More importantly, standardized assessments are out of context in that they fail to address the uniqueness of each child and the uniqueness of their circumstances. By contrast, behavioural observation strategies represent an approach to assessment that focusses on the individual child within the various, specific contexts of home and preschool that the child is involved in.

BEHAVIOUR OBSERVATIONS: LINKING ASSESSMENT TO TEACHING

Behavioural observation comprises what infants and children do in natural contexts with parents and other significant persons. In addition to a concern for data that evaluates behaviour in relation to naturally occurring response antecedents and consequences, behavioural strategies emphasize the need for repeated measures across time and across settings. This multiple measures strategy reflects the theoretical premise that behaviour is largely controlled by environmental events and that, given the complexity of behaviour–environment interactions, a single measure will fail to indicate both variable and stable patterns of responding.

Where repeated measures of the same responses show a variable response frequency and/or topography, then this provides an opportunity for evaluating functional relationships between the environmental conditions that pertain when particular responding patterns are evident. From such data, stimuli that are associated with desirable responding (e.g. attention, smiling, vocalization, manipulation of objects) and with less desirable responding (e.g. resistance to food ingestion, screaming, self-stimulation) may be identified. Intervention may then involve changes to the physical and social features of the infant's environment that may promote adaptive responding.

Where repeated observation measures show stable response patterns that indicate non-adaptive behaviours then this assessment data will form the baseline against which to measure the effectiveness of an intervention designed to teach a new skill. Ballard and Medland (1986), for example, report such data from their work with a two and a half year old girl who showed developmental delays and autistic-like behaviours. They showed the child's parents and teachers strategies for helping the child interact appropriately with toys. Baseline measures in the home and in the preschool setting were at zero levels whereas following the intervention programme the data showed appropriate child responses in both settings.

Behavioural researchers, teachers and psychologists have consistently worked with, and successfully taught, infants and children who have the severest of physical, cognitive, social and multiple disabilities (e.g. Haring and Bricker, 1978; Sailor and Guess, 1983; Vincent *et al.*, 1980). Their theoretical model has emphasized the power of the environment, requiring assessment within the contexts that the child has to learn from and optimism that children will learn if we can only design their environments to meet their special needs. This conceptual position, together with the direct relation of assessment strategies and data to intervention strategies and evaluation data, offers positive features for assessment for early intervention. At the same time, behavioural approaches have some features that are potentially limiting factors for both assessment and intervention.

A major direction taken by the behavioural approach has been to develop an instructional technology for teaching skills to children and adults who have severe handicaps (Guess and Noonan, 1982). This instructional technology has emphasized task analysis, which involves a breakdown of skills into specific, component behaviours. Guess and Noonan agree with the observations of Liberty and Wilcox (1981, p. 1), who report on teachers 'trained to perform countless acts of reductionism on a variety of tasks' resulting in the '42-step analysis of shoe tying' and related, complex, technical approaches to instruction that are inappropriate, inoperable and unnecessary in many educational settings.

Such behavioural instruction has also tended to show greater concern with predetermined goals and task hierarchies than with the characteristics of the individual learner (Ballard, 1987). One result of this highly structured approach to instruction has been tight stimulus control resulting in the failure of newly learned responses to generalize to complex natural settings, a problem that has been particularly salient in behavioural language programmes (Spradlin and Siegel, 1982).

THE EMERGING INFLUENCE OF ECOLOGICAL APPROACHES

The behavioural focus on specific responses for assessment and instruction allows for precise, reliable measures and focused teaching goals. At the same time, behavioural assessment has often ignored the fact that a single response or behavioural skill is only a part of a child's complex repertoire, while behavioural interventions have often focused on teaching isolated skills without attention to the integrated and interrelated nature of human behaviour (Voeltz and Evans, 1982; Willems, 1974). Also, the technology of instruction derived from behavioural principles does not include a rationale or systematic guidelines on what to teach children who have disabilities.

Closely related to the issue of what to teach is the issue of what to assess. Important developments in planning the curriculum content for persons who have disabilities have come from the concept of the 'criterion of ultimate function' (Brown, Nietupski and Hamre-Nietupski, 1976) which represents strategies for determining the skills and understandings that a specific individual will need in order to function as independently as possible in mainstream settings. As Guess and Noonan (1982) note, these strategies identify the important skills necessary for age-appropriate, functional interactions in the natural settings of home, school and community. They therefore represent an 'ecological inventory approach' (p. 8) that stresses the relationship between the child and the requirements of specific settings.

For the infant and preschool child, this ecological inventory approach focuses on 'the criteria of the next educational environment' (Vincent *et al.*, 1980) by providing ecological assessments of what should be taught for successful placement in mainstream preschool and subsequent school settings. This model emphasizes social and behavioural 'survival skills' such as compliance, attention, social interaction and following directions (Guess and Noonan, 1982, p. 8). For example, Rietveld (1983) planned to involve children from her early intervention project in mainstream preschool settings. She first assessed the mainstream setting and observed that selecting an activity was a significant skill relevant to effective engagement in these settings. She therefore taught the children in her project how to make choices between alternative preschool activities.

ASSESSMENT AS AN ECOLOGICAL SYSTEMS ANALYSIS

Bronfenbrenner's (1979) ecological model of human development suggests that assessment of the child should include evaluation of the family and consider issues such as the value system of the community (e.g. attitudes to children who have disabilities) and the impact of political-resource factors (e.g. government support and provision for mainstreaming). Such an ecological systems perspective also represents a transactional model of development in which biological impairment is not seen as a static impediment to developmental progress (Guralnick, 1982). A transactional approach stresses that development proceeds through reciprocal interactions between children and environments so that both the individual and their settings experience change.

One implication of a transactional model is that planned changes in the child's family, educational and related environments may radically alter interaction patterns with significant implications for child development and learning. Changed interactions may minimize or even overcome biologically based disabilities. Such a possibility brings into question the relevance of intelligence testing and related attempts to predict a child's future developmental achievements. A transactional model also casts doubt on the value of other forms of assessment that involve measuring behaviours away from the natural contexts in which child responses occur. Instead, a transactional perspective emphasizes assessments of children in the settings in which they live and with the persons with whom they interact. Such assessments include collecting information on how the participants in the child's family and related ecological systems perceive their own and the child's world. As Scott (1980) suggests, the term 'ecology' refers to the total context of behaviour. This not only includes the physical characteristics of the environment but also requires attention to attributes such as roles and social rules. Roles and social rules are subjective culture-bound perspectives, as are parent and teacher expectations, which also form part of the ecology of child development and learning (Wallace and Larsen, 1978).

If we are to include subjective data in assessments then there is need to address issues in the area of phenomenologically oriented knowledge. These issues include the idea that there is no final, objective 'truth' because reality differs from person to person, from parent to professional, and from administrator to teacher. Heshusius (1981) suggests that attempting to understand the perspectives of significant others is extremely practical because it increases awareness of alternative views and options for action, and can lead to clearer communication. Clear communication should be a major focus in assessments of infants and young children. This is because the infant's well-being is dependent on a range of others, in particular parents, mediating between the child and his or her social environment. Therefore, any planning designed to enhance developmental opportunities through early intervention programmes requires that parents, teachers and other professionals understand one anothers' expectations and goals.

The idea that an individual's expectations and assumptions are important aspects of the infant's environment has implications for the role of the psychologist or other person who is primarily responsible for assessment. Clearly, if a psychologist thinks mainly in terms of the factors limiting a child's development their assessments are likely to be predictive and pessimistic. On the other hand, if a psychologist rejects a 'test and predict' perspective and is oriented toward optimism and effective programming then enthusiasm is likely to be generated for developing responsive environments for the child.

An ecological perspective requires, therefore, that the psychologist examine his or her assumptions, concepts and cultural perspectives and attempts to evaluate how those ideas will impact on each child they work with. Such critical evaluation acknowledges that the psychologist becomes part of the child's and the family's ecological surroundings. The influence that the psychologist's cultural understanding and related ideas might have on the child's development, therefore, demands ongoing professional self-evaluation.

Assessment that is guided by such an ecological model is a process that recognizes the need to understand infant development and infant environment as interdependent. Ecological assessment is driven by an intention to change child behaviour and experiences rather than to simply compare a child's performance with a normative model. Ecological assessment, therefore, involves more than test responses and objective behaviour observa-

143

tions, and includes the perceptions and interpretations of the psychologist and of significant others in the infant's life. As Haywood (1977) suggests, it is 'time to return the intelligent observer to psychology, and to stop trying to reduce the psychologist to a mere recorder of data that can then be referred to a computerized set of comparison norms' (p. 17).

Intelligent observation requires involvement with families across time. This means that the psychologist's work resembles participant observation (Smith, 1978; Jacob, 1987) and must include recognition that empirical strategies provide only one kind of scientific data (Astman, 1984). Accepting both qualitative and quantitative as valid assessment data is, therefore, an important step toward ecological assessment. The techniques and skills required for such an approach to assessment would include observational strategies similar to those used in ethnography. Wolcott (1982) describes the ethnographer as a 'research instrument' with a commitment to spending an adequate amount of time in the field, to gathering information using multiple strategies, and to describing and interpreting rather than rendering judgements. For example, parent and teacher views form part of the ecosystem of home and preschool which includes affect, physical arrangements, daily activities and surrounding social conditions. To access some of this information, Voeltz and Evans (1983) recommend simple anecdotal notes in the form of a daily teacher and parent diary or home–school notebook that would monitor behaviours across time and settings. Such notes include objective records of behaviour and also notes on the child's, parents' and teacher's overall reactions (such as mood, compliance, enjoyment) to ongoing programmes. From such information, the psychologist, parent and teacher together may develop and test hypotheses to explain both positive and negative changes in a child's responding.

Zigmond and Silverman (1984) refer to such assessment strategies as 'informal' processes which are situation-specific and non-standardized. They suggest that they are more likely to contribute to programme planning and evaluation than are tests that are unrelated to the child's experiences or curriculum. For some psychologists the term 'informal' is interpreted as meaning less 'scientific'. Tests, on the other hand, are more likely to be viewed as properly scientific. Such a view ignores the fact that infant tests are largely lacking in construct validity and lack norms for children who have disabilities (Fuchs *et al.*, 1987). On the other hand, there is an extensive research base in psychology that would allow the psychologist to design and interpret alternative assessment strategies using observation methods, interview data and self-report data from parents, teachers and others. When carefully, systematically and explicitly based on appropriate theory and research, such assessment can have both construct and ecological validity and will therefore be more 'scientific' than so-called 'formal' testing.

Having reviewed various approaches to assessment for infants who have disabilities, the present chapter suggests that ecological theory can guide the development of assessment strategies that acknowledge the transactional nature of infant development and address the complexity of infant learning in social contexts. The final section of this chapter will outline procedures that would contribute to such an assessment. Before undertaking such a summary it is relevant to comment on the team approach to assessment as one strategy for coping with the varied and complex needs of infants who have disabilities.

THE ASSESSMENT TEAM FOR MULTIPLE DISABILITIES

Sailor and Guess (1983) suggest that because infants and children who have severe disabilities display delicate health conditions and a number of developmental, sensory and motor delays, then assessment and early intervention must include a coordinated effort by professionals and parents. Sailor and Guess advocate a transdisciplinary approach which integrates programme goals and objectives from various disciplines and professionals. The essence of this approach is that each team person willingly shares information and skills so that various interventions with the child can occur simultaneously. To achieve this it is necessary for team members to educate one another from the perspective of their information and skills and to accept that they can teach others (including parents) to implement procedures and skills that have usually been the responsibility of particular professionals. Coordination of this multiple effort (with pediatrician, nutritionist, physical therapist, psychologist, parents etc.) is through one team member who becomes programme facilitator. Sailor and Guess suggest that as the teacher is the professional who has most contact with the child, this person would often take on the facilitator role. They also emphasize that the transdisciplinary team model should be a flexible approach that responds to the needs of individual children and their families. For example, not every team member may be needed for every case.

This latter point is important as Fewell (1983b) has cautioned against the notion that 'more is better' in a team approach, citing research that suggests no superiority for a coordinated team over less formal arrangements. Nevertheless, there may still be value in one person ensuring that the various professionals involved in a case relate effectively with the parents and with one another.

ASSESSMENT FOR EARLY INTERVENTION: SOME BASIC REQUIREMENTS

From the preceding review a number of issues emerge that may be used to guide thinking about the kind of assessment strategies most likely to contribute to an intervention programme.

Assessment should focus on adaptive behaviour

Assessment that is relevant for teaching should evaluate actual performance on tasks relevant to an intervention programme. This involves recording data on children as they engage in actual motor, social, communication and language tasks, rather than scoring their performance on psychometric tests. Using tests to make inferences about potential performance cannot be justified when a more ecologically valid assessment can be achieved by observing actual performance in the area of interest. Assessment, therefore, must move away from diagnostic testing in the psychologist's office to measures of actual infant performance in meaningful social contexts. This would involve a move away from normative comparisons to evaluating the kinds of behaviours actually involved in teaching.

A developmental checklist such as the Portage Guide to Early Education (Bluma *et al.*, 1978) can provide a guide to the skill areas that require evaluation through observation, and can be a useful summary device for recording a general overview of skill levels (e.g. Ballard and Sinclair, 1981). Nevertheless, such guides are neither precise enough (Brown and York, 1974) nor conceptually appropriate (Sailor and Guess, 1983, and earlier discussion in this chapter) for designing a curriculum for individuals. Instead, assessment of each child and of the settings they live in requires a detailed observation using various observation strategies (e.g. Genishi, 1982; Irwin and Bushnell, 1980; Sackett, 1978). The focus of observational assessment should be guided by current research in each relevant area such as communication (e.g. Barnett, 1987; Peck and Schuler, 1986) or social skills (e.g. Donnellan and Neel, 1986; Guralnick, 1982; Guess and Siegel-Causey, 1985).

Assessment Should Be Based On Repeated Sampling Of Behaviour

If a child fails to respond to a test item it may mean that the concept or action is not part of their response repertoire. However, it may also mean that the child has the action or information but cannot recall it at that time. It may also be the case that, in the particular circumstances such as the language or communication style used, the setting, or the persons involved, the child may fail to use a strategy that in other settings is used effectively. This is an experience that parents have been telling psychologists about for years.

Assessment of performance on a single occasion is generally a poor predictor of behaviour at other times in other settings (Epstein, 1980; Clarke and Clarke, 1973). Assessment should, therefore, involve repeated measures in order to adequately and reliably sample infant skills. Ballard and Crooks (1984), for example, showed that the social interactions of both randomly selected and socially withdrawn children in a preschool setting varied considerably from day to day, so that assessment on one occasion did not provide accurate data on level of social behaviours.

147

Repeated measures assessment can form the baseline against which to evaluate a teaching intervention. Observational assessment as an ongoing, day-by-day activity provides detailed information on a child's response to intervention and can ensure that unsuccessful teaching or other intervention strategies are promptly identified and changed.

Assessment Should Be Ecologically Valid

An ecological approach stresses the complex interrelationships and interdependencies between children and their environments (Gump, 1975; Carlson, Scott and Eklund, 1980). Ecological assessment involves 'data taken across environments, persons, curricular areas and instructional conditions' (Bradley and Howe, 1980 p. 9) so that the infant's responses are evaluated across various stimulus conditions and social circumstances. The concept of ecological assessment is basically concerned with how meaningful particular assessment data are in terms of the child's real life experiences and needs. This must include recognition of the child's cultural background and experience.

Ecological assessment requires that children are assessed where they normally live and with the people they usually interact with. The emphasis is on evaluating actual learning behaviours, rather than on making inferences and projections from tests, developmental checklists and interviews. This does not preclude the value of novelty – indeed, testing the child's reaction to a change in the environment, materials or persons can be a valuable procedure for developing new experiences for the child. However, undertaking such evaluation in natural settings provides additional data on parent and teacher reaction to such materials and procedures.

Ecological assessment involves a functional approach in which evaluation is made of what the child needs to know in order to adjust and learn in a present environment, or in an environment in which it is planned to involve the child at some future time (Zigmond and Miller, 1986). Such an approach involves assessment of the features and demands of specific environments and then assessment of what the child needs to learn in order to function effectively in those settings. Assessment should also indicate what changes can be made to the environment (both physical and social arrangements) that may enhance child adaptation and experience. Assessment should proceed using repeated observations and anecdotal diary records, and psychologist and teacher-made curriculum-referenced assessments. Such assessment procedures allow adaptation to the unique characteristics of a particular child and family, and represent the first steps in promoting skills across various instructional domains.

Parents and Teachers Should be Meaningfully Involved In Assessment

Research to date suggests that the greatest gains in child development occur when intervention is initiated within the first two years of the child's life and where parents are meaningfully involved from the beginning (Sailor and Haring, 1978). Ecological assessment includes the psychologist developing a collaborative partnership with parents and teachers where the understandings, skills and preferences of each participant are equally valued and openly shared (Bailey, 1987; Russell, 1983). Involvement with parents and teachers must include sensitivity to cultural, ethnic, and value differences. Interactions with parents should also recognize that parents will differ in their views on the parental role. Some may resent 'professionalization' of their role if they perceive pressures to undertake teaching and advocacy as inappropriate for them and their approach to family interactions (Allen and Hudd, 1987; Voeltz, 1984).

Initial interviews should clearly tell parents and teachers that the information and perspectives they have on the child are respected and valued, and that they are viewed as part of the assessment team. Within such a partnership relationship, guidelines for identifying and prioritizing intervention goals are essential. Sulzer-Azaroff and Mayer (1977, p. 42) present useful procedures which require answers to such questions as the importance of the goal to the child and to significant others (parents, teacher), whether the goal is likely to be maintained in the client's natural settings, and evaluation of the time and effort required of the child and others to achieve the goal. Using such an approach can help the psychologist, parent and teacher make explicit their ethical, value and resource concerns during goal selection for early intervention.

ASSESSMENT SHOULD ADDRESS THE DYNAMIC NATURE OF INFANT DEVELOPMENT

Assessment for intervention must take into account the dynamic features of child developmental processes which include how children influence those who influence them; how intervention might correspond to the child's current developmental status; and how the child becomes an 'agent, shaper and selector', effectively fitting skills to setting demands or changing the setting to better meet personal attributes (Kendall, Lerner and Craighead, 1984). These authors emphasize that socialization is reciprocal and that, for example, children with different biologically determined temperaments interact differently with adults and may be perceived differently by them. A critical issue for assessment is the need to recognize such circular functions and to avoid identifying problems or strengths within only one part of a reciprocal system. For this reason a family systems perspective represents a valuable model for analyzing the needs of the family that has a child with a disability (Vincent and Salisbury, 1988).

Viewing the child as a processor involves understanding that at different times specific experiences have different meanings, depending on the child's current physical, cognitive, social and emotional development. Also, if the child is viewed as an interactive-reactive processor then it is equally important to assess what the child is processing and interacting with at various times. For example, the affective climate of the family varies according to internal and external circumstances (e.g. parental employment), and a child's responses must be evaluated in the light of such environmental contexts at different times. From this perspective, an understanding of variability in developmental processes evident in children, who do not have disabilities, and their families, would help ensure that assessment and intervention takes into account the usual range of experiences in age-associated cognitions, behaviours and developmental changes. It is often helpful for both parents and professionals to note that consistent child compliance and smooth learning curves are not realistic experiences or expectations for any child.

Assessment Should Be Credible And Meaningful To The Consumer

Assessment data contributes to early intervention only to the extent that it is understood and valued by parents, teachers and others who are caring for the child and implementing teaching programmes. If assessment of the infant is undertaken in a clinical setting away from parents and teacher, and if the data differs from their experience or is presented in technical terms that they cannot understand, then such information is unlikely to be used by parents, caregivers or teachers in programme design or evaluation. Parents and teachers should be encouraged to assist with the assessment of infants and young children and to make their own judgments and comments on how sensible and relevant the strategies are for their child and their needs.

Assessment And Teaching Should Proceed Together

Parents and teachers want to know what they can do to help the child. Assessment outcomes are often not credible or meaningful to parents or teachers because assessment data alone does not provide adequate guidelines for action. Very often too much time is committed to assessment tasks which then require further time for translation into teaching goals and strategies. This suggests the need to rethink not just assessment data but also assessment processes. One solution is to see teaching as assessment. If we see teaching as a responsive, hypothesis testing, trial-and-error process, then setting out to actually teach the infant something may be an optimum assessment strategy. The goal of early intervention is to support parents and to assist each individual family to identify strategies which are acceptable to them and which will optimize developmental opportunities for their child. Working with parents in their home to actually teach the infant something will help reveal child skills and needs and will identify parent skills and related environmental supports for learning within the cultural, value and resource circumstances of the family. A careful analysis of running record type accounts of such teaching sessions, in which both parents and professionals show one another how they engage with the child, will provide quantitative, qualitative and ecologically valid data. At the same time such sessions contribute to the establishment of a genuine partnership between parent and professional. Such a partnership may help identify critical skills (Guess and Noonan, 1982) which are behaviours likely to have multiple positive collateral outcomes (Voeltz and Evans, 1982). For example, teaching a child to roll a ball may include cognitive, social, communicative and affective learning and involve parents, siblings and others in new interactions.

The Results Of Assessment Should Maximize The Chances Of Effective Intervention For Each Child

If parents, teachers and others are to commit themselves to an intervention programme it is important for assessment data to be communicated in terms which reflect optimism that learning will occur as a result of their efforts. Such optimism is unlikely to be engendered by predictive statements of 'potential' based on normative comparisons. On the other hand, repeated observation data and anecdotal records of meaningful behaviours in natural settings can indicate emergent skills and the contexts most likely to lead to repetition and development of functional adaptive behaviours. Such a record of learning is likely to encourage optimism regarding future learning. Also, showing a parent or teacher how their infant orients to specific sounds or to a novel stimulus will be more meaningful for them than reporting a test score or checklist summary. Listening to parents and helping them to evaluate and implement their own ideas ideas can further extend support for their efforts while at the same time communicating belief in the plasticity and open-endedness of development.

SUMMARY: EVALUATING CHILD DEVELOPMENT AND LEARNING IN CONTEXT

This chapter has presented a case for assessing young children as they interact with parents and with related persons and environments in which they develop and learn. It has been suggested that assessment strategies can be derived from both quantitative and qualitative observation methodologies and that these observation procedures may be undertaken and interpreted from ecological and systems theory perspectives. These perspectives involve recognition of phenomenological issues including family culture and value identity. Detailed observation records of teaching undertaken by both parents and professionals have been suggested as an optimal assessment strategy with multiple outcome data that will help ensure that early intervention is undertaken with a minimum of delay.

A central theme for the chapter has been a belief in the plasticity of development, recognizing with Bloom (1982) that human potential is much greater than that shown in our assessments or realized by our educational methods. A transactional perspective on child development rejects the predictive outcomes of testing as representing an inappropriately static model and a futile enterprise. Instead, assessment efforts should be directed toward understanding each child's development as a complex, ongoing, reciprocal, interactional process that parents, teachers and psychologists can learn from and continue to influence.

To reiterate the main points developed in this chapter:

1. Assessment should focus on adaptive behaviours.
2. Assessment should be based on repeated sampling of behaviours.
3. Assessment should be ecologically valid.
4. Parents and teachers should be meaningfully involved in assessment.
5. Assessment should address the dynamic nature of infant development.
6. Assessment should be credible and meaningful to the consumer.
7. Assessment and teaching should proceed together.
8. The results of assessment should maximize the chances of effective intervention for each child.

153

REFERENCES

Allen, D. A. and Hudd, S. S. (1987) 'Are We Professionalizing Parents? Weighing the Benefits and Pitfalls,' *Mental Retardation*, 25, 133–139.

Anastasi, A. (1976) *Psychological Testing* (4th ed.), Macmillan Publishing Co., New York.

Astman, J. A. (1984) 'Special Education as a Moral Enterprise,' *Learning Disability Quarterly*, 7, 299–308.

Bailey, D. B. (1987) 'Collaborative Goal-setting with Families: Resolving Differences in Values and Priorities for Services,' *Topics in Early Childhood Education*, 7(2), 59–71.

Ballard, K. D. (1987) 'The Limitations of Behavioural Approaches to Teaching: Some Implications for Special Education,' *The Exceptional Child*, 34, 1–16.

Ballard, K. D. (1988) 'Toward the Non-restrictive Environment,' *The Exceptional Child Monograph No.1*, 7–18.

Ballard, K. D. and Crooks, T. (1984) 'Videotape Modelling for Children with Low Levels of Social Interaction and Low Peer Involvement in Play,' *Journal of Abnormal Child Psychology*, 12, 95–109.

Ballard, K. D. and Medland, J. (1986) 'Collateral Effects from Teaching Attention, Imitation and Toy Interaction Behaviours to a Developmentally Handicapped Child,' *Child and Family Behavior Therapy*, 7, 47–60.

Ballard, K. D. and Sinclair, P. (1981) *Developmental profile (from birth to six years) Portage Early Educational Programme*, NFER-Nelson, Berkshire.

Barnett, J. (1987) 'Research on Language and Communication in Children who have Severe Handicaps: A Review and Some Implications for Intervention,' *Educational Psychology*, 7, 117–128.

Bayley, N. (1969) *Manual for the Bayley Scales of Infant Development*, Psychological Corporation, New York.

Bloom, B. S. (1982) 'The Future of Educational Research,' *Educational Researcher*, 11 (8), 12–13.

Bluma, S. M., Shearer, M. S., Frohman, A. H., and Hillard, J. M. (1978) *Portage Guide to Early Education* (rev. ed.), Cooperative Educational Service Agency, Portage, Wisconsin.

Bradley, C., McD., and Howe, C. E. (1980) 'Administrative Issues in Evaluation of Exceptionality,' *Exceptional Education Quarterly*, 1, 1–12.

Bronfenbrenner, U. (1979) *The Ecology of Human Development: Experiments by Nature and Design*, Harvard University Press, Cambridge, MA.

Brown, L. and York, R. (1974) 'Developing Programs for Severely Handicapped Students: Teacher Training and Classroom Instruction', *Focus on Exceptional Children, 6,* 1–11.

Brown, L., Nietupski, J., and Hamre-Nietupski, S. (1976) 'Criterion of Ultimate Functioning,' in M. A. Thomas (ed.), *Hey, Don't Forget About Me,* Council for Exceptional Children, Reston, VA pp. 2–15.

Carlson, C. I., Scott, M., and Eklund, S. M. (1980) 'Ecological Theory and Method for Behavioral Assessment,' *School Psychology Review, 9,* 75-82.

Cattell, P. (1940) *The Measurement of Intelligence of Infants and Young Children,* Psychological Corporation, New York.

Clarke, A. D. B. and Clarke, A. M. (1973) 'Assessment and Prediction,' in P. J. Mittler (ed.), *Assessment for Learning in the Mentally Handicapped,* Churchill Livingstone, London.

Collard, R. R. (1972) 'Review of the Bayley Scales of Infant Development,' in O. K. Buros (ed.), *The Seventh Mental Measurement Yearbook,* The Gryphone Press, New Jersey, pp. 727-729.

Donnellan, A.M. and Neel, R.S. (1986) 'New Directions in Educating Students with Autism,' in R.H. Horner, L.H. Meyer and H.D. Fredericks (eds.), *Education of Learners with Severe Handicaps: Exemplary Service Strategies,* Paul H. Brooks, Baltimore.

DuBose, R. F. (1982) 'Assessment of Severely Impaired Young Children: Problems and Recommendations,' in J. T. Nelsworth (ed.), *Assessment in Special Education,* Aspen, Rocville, Maryland, pp. 199–211.

Dunst, C. J. and Rheingrover, R. M. (1982) 'Discontinuity and Instability in Early Development: Implications for Assessment,' in J. T. Neisworth (ed.), *Assessment in Special Education,* Aspen, Rockville, Maryland.

Eippert, D. S. and Azen, S. P. (1978) 'A Comparison of Two Developmental Instruments in Evaluating Children with Down's Syndrome,' *Physical Therapy, 58,* 1066–1069.

Epstein, S. (1980) 'The Stability of Behaviour II: Implications for Psychological Research,' *American Psychologist, 35,* 790–806.

Fewell, R. R. (1983a) 'Assessing Handicapped Infants,' in S. G. Garwood and R. R. Fewell (eds), *Educating Handicapped Infants: Issues in Development and Intervention,* Aspen Publications, Rockville, Maryland, pp. 257-297.

Fewell, R. R. (1983b) 'The Team Approach to Infant Education,' in S. G. Garwood & R. R. Fewell (eds), *Educating Handicapped Infants: Issues in Development and Intervention,* Aspen Publications, Rockville, Maryland, pp. 299–322.

Fewell, R. R. (1984) 'Assessment of Preschool Handicapped Children,' *Educational Psychologist, 19,* 3, 172–179.

Frankeburg, W. K., Dobbs, J. B., and Fandal, A. W. (1967) *Denver Developmental Screening Test*, University of Colorado Medical Center.

Fuchs, D., Fuchs, L. S., Benowitz, S., and Barringer, K. (1987) 'Norm Referenced Tests: Are They Valid for Use with Handicapped Students?' *Exceptional Children*, 54, 263–271.

Fuchs, D., Fuchs, L. S., Power, M. H., and Dailey, A. M. (1985) 'Bias in the Assessment of Handicapped Children,' *American Educational Research Journal*, 22, 185–198.

Genishi, C. (1982) 'Observational Research Methods for Early Childhood Education,' in B. Spodek (ed.), *Handbook of Research in Early Childhood Education*, Free Press, New York, pp. 564–581.

Gentry, D. and Adams, G. (1978) 'A Curriculum-Based, Direct Intervention Approach to the Education of Handicapped Infants,' in N. G. Haring and D. Bricker (eds), *Teaching The Severely Handicapped, Vol. III*, American Association for the Education of the Severely/Profoundly Handicapped, Seattle, pp. 94–123.

Gesell, A. (1940) *The First Five Years of Life*, Harper, New York.

Gesell, A. and Amatruda, C. (1947) *Developmental Diagnosis*, Harper and Row, New York.

Griffiths, R. (1970) *The Abilities of Young Children*, Child Development Research Centre, London.

Guess, D. and Noonan, M. J. (1982) 'Curricula and Instructional Procedures for Severely Handicapped Students,' *Focus on Exceptional Children*, 14, 5, 1–12.

Guess, D. and Siegel-Causey, E. (1985) 'Behavioral Control and Education of Severely Handicapped Students: Who's Doing What to Whom? and Why?,' in D. Bricker and J. Fuller (eds), *Severe Mental Retardation: From Theory to Practice*, The Council for Exceptional Children, Reston, VA, pp. 456–500.

Gump, P. V. (1975) 'Ecological Psychology and Children,' in E. M. Hetherington (ed.), *Review of Child Development Research, Vol. 5*, University of Chicago Press, Chicago.

Gurnalnick, M. J. (1982) 'Mainstreaming Young Handicapped Children: A Public Policy and Ecological Systems Analysis,' in B. Spodek (ed), *Handbook of Research in Early Child–hood Education*, Free Press, New York.

Haring, W. G. and Bricker, D. D. (1978) *Teaching the Severely Handicapped (Vol. III)*, American Association for the Education of the Severely/Profoundly Handicapped, Seattle.

Haywood, H. C. (1977) 'Alternatives to Normative Assessment,' in P. Mittler (ed.), *Research to Practice in Mental Retardation, Vol. II*, Education and Training, University Park Press, Baltimore, pp. 11–18.

Heshusius, L. (1981) *Meaning in Life as Experienced by Persons Labeled Retarded in a Group Home: A Participant Observation Study*, Charles C. Thomas, Springfield, Illinois.

Hunt, J. McV. (1974) 'Psychological Assessment, Developmental Plasticity, and Heredity, with Implications for Early Intervention,' in G. J. Williams and S. Gordon (eds), *Clinical Child Psychology: Current Practices and Future Perspectives*, Behavioral Publications, New York, pp.119–141.

Irwin, D. M. and Bushnell, M. M. (1980) *Observational Strategies for Child Study*, Holt, Rinehart and Winston, New York.

Jacob, E. (1987) 'Qualitative Research Traditions: A Review,' *Review of Educational Research*, 57, 1–50.

Johnson, N. M. (1982) 'Assessment Paradigms and Atypical Infants: An Interventionist's Perspective,' in D. D. Bricker (ed.), *Intervention with At-risk and Handicapped Infants: From Research to Application*, University Park Press, Baltimore.

Kendall, P. C., Lerner, R. M., and Craighead, W. E. (1984) 'Human Development and Intervention in Childhood Psychopathology,' *Child Development*, 55, 71–82.

Liberty, K. and Wilcox, B. (1981) 'Forum: Slowing Down Learning,' *Association for the Severely Handicapped Newsletter*, 1, 2, 1–2.

Messick, S. (1983) 'Assessment of Children,' in P.H. Kessen, volume editor, *Vol. 1. History, Theory and Methods*, J. Wiley, New York, pp. 477-526.

Peck, C. A. and Schuler, A. L. (1986) 'Assessment of Social/ Communicative Behavior for Students with Autism and Severe Handicaps: The Importance of Asking the Right Question,' in T. Layton (ed.), *Language Intervention and Treatment of Autistic and Developmentally Disordered Children*, Charles C. Thomas, Columbus, OH.

Ramsay, M. and Fitzhardinge, P. M. (1977) 'A Comparative Study of Two Developmental Scales: The Bayley and the Griffiths,' *Early Human Development*, 1, 151–157.

Rietveld, C. M. (1983) 'The Training of Choice Behaviours in Down's Syndrome and Non-Retarded Preschool Children,' *Australia and New Zealand Journal of Developmental Disabilities*, 9, 75–83.

Russell, P. (1983) 'The Parents' Perspective of Family Needs and How to Meet Them,' in P. Mittler and H. McConachie (eds), *Parents, Professionals and Mentally Handicapped People: Approaches to Partnership*, Croom Helm, London, pp. 47–61.

Sackett, G. P. (1978) *Observing Behaviour: Vol. 1. Theory and Applications in Mental Retardation*, University Park Press, Baltimore.

Sailor, W. and Guess, D. (1983) *Severely Handicapped Students: An Instructional Design*, Houghton Mifflin Co., Dallas.

Sailor, W. and Haring, N. G. (1978) 'Progress in the Education of the Severely/Profoundly Handicapped,' in N. G. Haring and D. D. Bricker (eds), *Teaching the Severely Handicapped (Vol. III)*, American Association for the Education of the Severely/Profoundly Handicapped, Seattle, pp. 47–61.

Scott, M. (1980) 'Ecological Theory and Methods for Research in Special Education,' *Journal of Special Education, 14*, 279–293.

Sheehan, R. (1982) 'Infant Assessment: A Review and Identification of Emergent Trends,' in D. Bricker (ed.), *Intervention with At-risk and Handicapped Infants: From Research to Application*, University Park Press, Baltimore.

Simeonsson, R. J., Huntington, G. S. and Parse, S. A. (1980) 'Assessment of Children with Severe Handicaps: Multiple Problems — Multivariate Goals,' *Journal of the Association for the Severely Handicapped, 5*, 1, 55–72.

Smith, L. M. (1978) 'An Evolving Logic of Participant Observation, Educational Ethnography and Other Case Studies,' in L. S. Shulman (ed), *Review of Research in Education, Vol. 6*, F. E. Peacock, Itasca, Illinois, pp. 316–377.

Spradlin, J. E. and Siegel, G. M. (1982) 'Language Training in Natural and Clinical Environments,' *Journal of Speech and Hearing Disorders, 47*, 2–6.

Stratford, B. (1985) 'Learning and Knowing: The Education of Down's Syndrome Children,' in D. Lane and B. Stratford (eds), *Current Approaches to Down's Syndrome*, Holt, Rinehart and Winston, London, pp. 149–166.

Sulzer-Azaroff, B. and Mayer, G. R. (1977) *Applying Behavior Analysis Procedures with Children and Youth*, Holt, Rinehart andWinston, New York.

Taylor, S. J., Racing, J., Knoll, J., and Lutfiyya, Z. (1986) *The Non-Restrictive Environment: A Resource Manual on Community Integration for People with the Most Severe Disabilities*, Community Integration Project, Center on Human Policy, Syracuse University, Syracuse, New York.

Uzgiris, I. C. and Hunt, J. McV. (1975) *Assessment in Infancy: Ordinal Scales of Psychological Development*, University of Illinois Press, Urbana, Illinois.

Vincent, L. J., Salisbury. C., Walter, G., Brown, P., Gruenwald, L. J., and Powers, M. (1980) 'Program Evaluation and Curriculum Development in Early Childhood/Special Education: Criteria of the Next Environment,' in W. Sailor, B. Wilcox, and L. Brown (eds.), *Methods of Instruction for Severely Handicapped Students*, Paul H. Brooks, Baltimore.

Vincent, L.J. and Salisbury, C.L. (1988) 'Changing Economic and Social Influences on Family Involvement', *Topics in Early Childhood Special Education, 8,*(1), 48–59.

Voeltz, L. M. (1984) 'Review of The School and Home Enrichment Program for Severely Handicapped Children (R. P. Hawkins, L. K. McGinnis, B. J. Bienick, D. M. Timmons, D. B. Eddy and J. D. Cone, Research Press, 1983, Champaign, Illinois),' *Child and Family Behavior Therapy, 6,* 79–82.

Voeltz, L. M. and Evans, I. M. (1982). 'The Assessment of Behavioural Interrelationships in Child Behaviour Therapy,' *Behavioural Assessment, 4,* 131–165.

Voeltz, L. M. and Evans, I. M. (1983) 'Educational Validity: Procedures to Evaluate Outcomes in Programs for Severely Handicapped Learners,' *The Journal of the Association for the Severely Handicapped, 8,* 3–15.

Wallace, G. and Larsen, S. C. (1978) *Educational Assessment of Learning Problems: Testing for Teaching,* Allyn and Bacon Inc., Boston.

Willems, E.P. (1974) 'Behavioural Technology and Behavioural Ecology,' *Journal of Applied Behaviour Analysis, 7,* 151–165.

Wolcott, H. F. (1982) 'Mirrors, Models and Monitors: Educator Adaptations of the Ethnographic Innovation,' in G. Spindler (ed.), *Doing the Ethnography of Schooling,* Holt, Rinehart and Winston, New York, pp.68–95.

Yang, R. K. and Bell, R. G. (1975) 'Assessment of Infants,' in P. McReynolds (ed), *Advances in Psychological Assessment (Vol. 3),* Jossey Bass, San Francisco, pp. 137–185.

Zelazo, P. R. (1982) 'Alternative Assessment Procedures for Handicapped Infants and Toddlers: Theoretical and Practical Issues,' in D. D. Bricker (ed.), *Intervention with At-risk and Handicapped Infants: From Research to Application,* University Park Press, Baltimore, pp. 107–128.

Zigmond, N. and Miller, S.E. (1986) 'Assessment for Instructional Planning,' *Exceptional Children, 52,* 501–509

Zigmond, N. and Silverman, R. (1984) 'Informal Assessment for Program Planning and Evaluation in Special Education,' *Educational Psychologist, 19,* 163–171.

7 ASSESSMENT-CURRICULUM SYSTEMS FOR EARLY CHILDHOOD/SPECIAL EDUCATION

Angela Notari, Kristine Slentz and Diane Bricker

INTRODUCTION

The focus of this chapter is on curricula for Early Childhood/ Special Education. Curriculum, or the content of instruction, is a critical element of the intervention process. We believe, however, that curriculum is but one element of a larger system, in which assessment, intervention and evaluation procedures are closely interconnected. The quality of the linkage between these elements plays a critical role in the functioning of an effective early intervention programme.

In this chapter, our approach is to view curricula within the larger context of a programme's assessment procedures. Discussions have been broadened to include information on the programmatic implications of assessment instruments and on procedures enabling the linkage between assessment and curricula.

DEFINITIONS

Assessment

Assessment is defined as obtaining entry or baseline information. Assessment is primarily a process of measurement (Hamilton and Swan, 1981), the quality of which is dependent upon the selection of an appropriate instrument designed to serve a specific purpose. Early childhood assessment instruments take many forms but serve one of three major purposes in intervention programmes: screening, diagnostic or instructional programming (Sheehan, 1982).

Screening, diagnostic and programmatic assessment can be viewed as the collection of increasingly specific information. At the most global level, screening is intended to identify children in need of further, more comprehensive assessment. Screening assessments are brief and economical to administer, and designed to answer the general question, 'Is there a problem?'

The goal of screening is to test efficiently and cost effectively large groups of children to identify those few who require more extensive assessment. Well known examples of screening instruments are the Apgar Scoring System (Apgar, 1953) and the Denver Developmental Screening Test (Frankenburg *et al.*, 1975).

Once a problem or delay in development is identified, the next step in the assessment process is to confirm the presence or absence of a specific problem (Sheehan, 1982). Screening instruments cannot adequately serve this purpose, since they do not provide the detailed information necessary to pinpoint a specific syndrome or dysfunction (Johnson, 1982). To accomplish this goal, diagnostic tests are needed that assess in detail a child's skills and abilities in the area or areas where global problems have been detected. The purpose of diagnostic tests is to answer the question 'What is the exact nature of the problem?'. Diagnostic assessment is most often conducted and interpreted by trained specialists and is, therefore, more expensive and lengthy than screening. Results of diagnostic assessments are used to qualify children as eligible for special services and for referral to appropriate agencies. Examples of diagnostic tests include the Bayley Scales of Infant Development (Bayley, 1969) and karyotype tests for chromosomal disorders.

Both screening and diagnostic assessments compare the performance of the individual child being tested to the performance or status of normative groups. This type of test is known as norm-referenced, because each child's score is evaluated against norms derived from testing a large standardization sample. The standardization samples are developed to be representative of the population of children in a certain area (e.g. USA) and thus include a cross-section of important demographic variables (age, gender, SES). Results of norm-referenced tests are typically reported as age norms, percentiles, or standardized scores.

Neither screening nor diagnostic assessments are designed to provide information relevant to the purpose of instructional programming. There are a number of technical and pragmatic problems inherent in using norm-referenced test items to guide the development of instructional content in early intervention programmes. The development of individual education plans (IEPs) requires a qualitatively different type of information than is generated by tests designed for other purposes (Garwood, 1982). For example, items on norm-referenced tests are chosen to discriminate between children and not for instructional appropriateness (see also Chapter 5 by Heath and Levin).

A third type of assessment, programmatic assessment, is designed to address specifically the need to obtain educationally relevant information and provide guidance in the development of instructional programmes. Programmatic assessment serves at least three functions (Bricker and Littman, 1982). This assessment process provides information for the generation of individual educational plans (IEPs), allows parents to compare their objectives for the child with interventionists' objectives and generates data for group programme evaluation. The type of assessment most compatible with the functions and purpose of instructional programming is one that compares a child's performance not to other children, but rather to a specified criterion or mastery level. This type of test is known as a criterion-referenced assessment.

The development of criterion-referenced tests for infants and young children, however, has created problems. First, some intervention programmes developed narrow instruments for specific purposes, limiting the utility of such instruments for other programmes (Fewell, 1983). Second, and more seriously, the majority of criterion-referenced instruments were developed using selected items from various norm-referenced instruments (Bailey, 1983; Johnson, 1982). This practice invalidates any age equivalencies, especially considering the loss of standardized procedures in criterion-referenced test administration. Third, very few criterion-referenced tests provide reliability and/or validity data (Bricker, 1989). Although the content of criterion-referenced tests may be more appropriate to intervention targets, change in a child's scores over time may reflect instability of the instrument instead of child progress.

Curriculum-based assessments are a direct application of criterion-referenced assessment strategies to instructional content. Assessment and curricular content are coordinated to address the same skills and abilities. The assessment measure provides information directly relevant to programming, and the success of intervention efforts are evaluated by subsequent administrations of the same measure. The quality of the curriculum-assessment package is dependent upon the quality of the assessment and curriculum components.

Curriculum

The most important purpose of programmatic assessment in early intervention settings is that of providing information for designing interventions (Dunst and Rheingrover, 1981; Slentz, 1986). A critical element of intervention is the curriculum component which delineates the content of instruction, as well as the choice of teaching strategies (Bailey, Jens, and Johnson, 1983). Usually curriculum is thought of as a series of activities and experiences organized to facilitate the attainment of specified educational goals, through implemented teaching procedures (Bricker, 1989; Dunst, 1981).

An aspect that strongly influences curriculum decisions is the interventionist's ideas about the nature of development (Schwartz and Robinson, 1982). Historically, three major philosophical perspectives, Romanticism, Cultural Transmission and Dialectism have influenced the formulation of three major models of development which serve as the basis for most educational practices in Western society (Dunst, 1981; Stevens and King, 1976).

Romanticism, exemplified by the philosophy of Jean-Jacques Rousseau, emphasizes the intrinsic potential for optimal development to occur, given a healthy environment. Development, viewed as genetically determined, occurs primarily through maturation. Studies of child development, such as those by Gesell, focused on the observation of behaviours thought to reflect internal maturational processes. Major developmental milestones are described, and serve as the basis for assessment and curricula.

The educational emphasis is on the self-directedness of learning within a non-oppressive, and enriched environment. This method is characteristic of the child-centered, traditional nursery school approach.

Although successfully implemented in preschool models designed for normal children, the use of self-directed, experiential approaches may be of concern when applied to children with special needs. Because of the special learning needs that accompany many handicapping conditions, these children need individual support and guidance.

The Cultural Transmission or Empirical Perspective, as exemplified by the philosophy of John Locke, emphasizes the role of the environment. Development, viewed as an additive accumulation of independent skills, is culturally determined. A major emphasis is placed on direct teaching using behavioural techniques based on principles derived from Skinner's theory of learning. Skills are taught through the manipulation of environmental stimuli and children are rewarded for emitting culturally desired behaviours. A variation of this approach is social learning theory, which emphasizes learning through imitation.

Programmed learning or direct instruction models, such as DISTAR (Bereiter and Englemann, 1966), have been successfully used with socially disadvantaged preschool children in the United States. Problems associated with direct instruction models are the lack of generalization to daily settings of skills learned in contrived situations, and the instructional dependency generated by training children to respond primarily to external cues provided by the adult (Guess and Seigel-Causey, 1983).

The Dialectical perspective views development as an ongoing, dynamic interaction between organism and environment. Knowledge is actively constructed by the child through exploration of the environment. The constructivist approach, postulated primarily by Jean Piaget, conjoins John Dewey's view of the role of education as facilitating the child's interactions with the environment.

The curricular emphasis from the dialectic perspective is on the process of learning, rather than on the product, and children are encouraged to take the initiative to explore and to experiment with materials. Piagetian-based curricula such as those developed by Kamii and DeVries (1978), Forman and Hill (1984) and by Hofmann, Banet and Weikart (1979) in the United States, and by the British Infant School Movement in England have been used with normal and environmentally at-risk children (Franklin and Biber, 1977).

More recently, the ecological perspective of development has provided a broad framework in which the organism-environment interactions are considered in relationship to societal and cultural systems (Bronfenbrenner, 1979). The ecological perspective has stimulated early intervention efforts to focus on the broad issues of infant-caregiver interaction, family involvement, and social support services (Dunst, 1986). The curricular emphasis is on the functioning in everyday, real-life situations and settings (Bricker, 1989; Hobbs, 1975). Skills taught are critical to development, but also functional in increasing the child's ability to cope with daily environmental demands. Instruction is activity-based, as it takes place within activities and settings that are part of the child's daily life experience (Bricker, 1986).

The ecological approach has been implemented in programmes for young children with handicaps, as well as youngsters whose development is at risk due to environmental and/or biologic factors. The Early Intervention Program at the University of Oregon in the United States, and at the Hester Adrian Research Centre at Manchester University in England are examples of ecologically based intervention efforts.

Linking Assessment and Curriculum

Although there is growing interest in linking programmatic assessment and curricula, many early intervention personnel view assessment and intervention processes as separate, with little conceptual or practical coordination. Assessment procedures or tools administered when the child enters the programme are often screening and diagnostic assessments. The outcome data are useful for placement or for describing the child's general repertoire. However, too frequently these data do not provide relevant information for the development of Individualized Education Plans (IEPs) or designing daily instructional activities (curricula).

Because experience has led interventionists to have little expectation that programmatically useful information will be forthcoming from the assessment process, curricular activities often reflect a weak relationship to the assessment strategy used. To develop the content of instruction, interventionists select items from a specific curriculum or more likely choose items from a variety of curricula. The choice of these items and of instructional content is made without benefit of accurate, comprehensive information on children's behavioural repertoires and without benefit of guidance on appropriate educational targets for intervention.

Until recently there has been a dearth of measurement tools and curricular materials that lend themselves to coordinated efforts (Johnson and Beauchamp, 1987). The acknowledgement that screening and diagnostic assessment do not yield programme relevant information and the need to link programme assessment and intervention is beginning to produce a variety of assessment and curricular materials that lend themselves to coordinated assessment and intervention efforts. These assessment-curriculum systems are generally called curriculum-based assessment. Assessment tools that yield information directly useful for the development of IEPs and instructional programmes offer an alternative that links assessment and curricula. In the present chapter we refer to these linked assessment-curriculum packages as assessment-curriculum systems.

REVIEW OF ASSESSMENT-CURRICULUM SYSTEMS

The premise underlying curriculum-based assessment systems is that assessment and intervention should not be considered as separate procedures, but as complementary aspects of a unique system. The purpose of creating a link between assessment and intervention content is to assure that the information generated by the assessment tool will be of relevance to the development of curricular content. Evaluation should also be considered a fundamental part of a linked system. Space limitations preclude including this phase, but for a discussion of how evaluation links to assessment and intervention see Bricker (1989).

Assessment is a key element to programming. Assessment items need to reflect the curricular content of the intervention programme (Bailey, 1983) and represent skills which can serve as a basis for the formulation of educationally relevant goals (Bagnato, Neisworth, and Capone, 1986). Educational goals contained in the curriculum should allow an easy reference back to the assessment component so that child progress may be monitored on a regular basis.

The overall effectiveness of the system relies on the quality of the linkage between assessment and curriculum as well as the qualities of the individual components. Linkage procedures should be direct and easy to implement. The assessment component should yield valid and reliable information on the child's level of functioning; the curriculum should focus on developmentally important skills which are functional for the child and which can be easily integrated within the child's daily activities; the subsequent assessment with the same instrument should provide objective and ecologically valid information to permit easy monitoring of child progress on a regular basis.

General Description

A number of assessment-curriculum systems are currently available for use with infants and young children. These systems vary considerably as to their organization, and format, and to the emphasis placed on their assessment, curriculum and evaluation components. The present review will describe ten instruments, all developed within the last 12 years. The basis for their inclusion in the review is that they provide guidelines and information for both assessment and programming. Table 1 lists these 10 assessment-curriculum systems accompanied by information on: 1) components that compose the system, 2) age range for whom the system is intended, 3) intended users, 4) intended purposes of the system, 5) theoretical framework that guided the development of the assessment and curricular materials, and 6) domains of behaviour included.

Supplementary information on each of the ten curricular-based assessment systems is provided below:

1. *The Portage Curriculum* (Bluma *et al.*, 1976) was designed for use with children from birth to six years of age. Originally developed to be used by parents in the home setting, it is divided into six developmental areas: Infant Stimulation, Socialization, Language, Self-Help, Cognitive, and Motor. The assessment component consists of a developmental checklist and is accompanied by a set of activity cards containing sets of activities for each item on the checklist.

Table 7.1: General information on the reviewed assessment-curriculum systems

TEST	COMPONENTS	POPULATION AGE RANGE	USERS	PURPOSES	THEORETICAL FRAMEWORK	DOMAINS
1. The Portage Guide to Early Education A. Bluma, M. Shearer, A. Frohman, and J. Hilliard, Portage WISC: The Portage Project, CESA 12, 1976: $50.00	Checklist Activity cards	Normal and handicapped children 0–6 years developmentally	Parents Teachers Paraprofessionals	Assessment Programming	Developmental Maturationist	Infant stimulation Socialization Language Motor Self-Help Cognition
2. Evaluation and Programming System (EPS-1) D. Bricker, D. Gentry, and E. Bailey, Eugene, OR: University of Oregon 1985: $30.00	Assessment manual Social-Communication Recording form Parent form Curriculum Software	Children 0–3 years developmentally	Early Intervention Direct Service Providers	Diagnosis Assessment Programming Evaluation	Developmental Functional	Fine motor Gross motor Self-Care Cognitive Social-Communication Social
3. Brigance Diagnostic Inventory of Early Development A. Brigance, North Billerica, MA: Curriculum Assessment, 1978: $50.00	Assessment manual Scoring booklets Graphs Materials (pictures)	Children 0–6 years developmentally	Teachers Paraprofessionals	Assessment Programming Record keeping Training resource	Developmental Maturationist	Psychomotor Self-Help Speech and language General knowledge and comprehension Early academic skills

Table 7.1: Continued

TEST	COMPONENTS	POPULATION AGE RANGE	USERS	PURPOSES	THEORETICAL FRAMEWORK	DOMAINS
4A. A Clinical and Educational Manual for Use with the Uzgiris and Hunt Scales of Infant Development C.J. Dunst, Baltimore, MD: University Park Press, 1980: $16.00	Assessment manual Record forms	Children functioning in the sensorimotor stage of development (0–18 months)	Professionals familiar with the Uzgiris and Hunt Scales	Assessment Programming Evaluation	Developmental Interactionist	Cognitive
4B. Infant Learning: A Cognitive-Linguistic Intervention Strategy C.J. Dunst, Allen, TX: DLM Teaching Resources, 1981: $27.00	Curriculum	Handicapped children functioning in the sensorimotor stage (0–18 months)	Early Interventionists	Programming	Developmental Interactionist Ecological	Cognitive Social-Communication
5. Hawaii Early Leaning Profile (HELP) S. Furuno et al, Palo Alto, CA: VORT 1979-Revised Ed., 1989: $21 (computer software excluded)	Checklist Profile (chart) Activity guide Computer software Curriculum guide for disabled parents	Handicapped children 0–3 years developmentally	Professionals Parents	Assessment Programming Evaluation	Developmental Maturationist/ interactionist	Cognitive Language Gross motor Fine motor Social-Emotional Self-Help

Table 7.1: Continued

TEST	COMPONENTS	POPULATION AGE RANGE	USERS	PURPOSES	THEORETICAL FRAMEWORK	DOMAINS
6. The Carolina Curriculum for Handicapped Infants and Infants at Risk W. Johnson-Martin, K. Jens, and S.H. Attenmeier, Baltimore, MD: Brookes, 1986: $29.95	Checklist Curriculum Individual activity sheets Progress chart	Children 0–24 months developmentally	Teachers Paraprofessionals	Assessment Programming Evaluation	Developmental Maturationist/ interactionist	Cognition Communication-language Social Self-Help Fine motor Gross motor
7. Arizona Basic Assessment and Curriculum for Young Children with Special Needs (ABACUS) J.M. McCarthy, K.A. Lund, C.S. Bos, and J. Blattke, Denver, CO: LOVE, 1985: $196.00	Screening assessment manual Communication sample Scoring booklet Curriculum Parent involvement and home teaching manual Evaluation manual	Handicapped children 2–5.5 years developmentally	Teachers	Screening Assessment Programming Evaluation	Developmental Functional Ecological	Body management Self-Care Communication Pre-Academic Socialization

Table 7.1: Continued

TEST	COMPONENTS	POPULATION AGE RANGE	USERS	PURPOSES	THEORETICAL FRAMEWORK	DOMAINS
8. Battelle Developmental Inventory J. Newborg, J.R. Stock, L. Wnek, J. Guidubaldi, and J. Svinicki, Allen, TX: DLM Teaching Resources, 1984: $185.00	Assessment manual Scoring booklet Profile Screening test Testing cards	Children 0–8 years	Professionals	Screening Assessment Programming Evaluation	Developmental Maturationist	Personal-Social Adaptive Motor Communication Cognitive
9. Developmental Programming for Infants and Young Children A) Early Intervention Developmental Programming and Profile (Revised version) S.S. Schafer and M.S. Moersch (Eds), Ann Arbor: University of Michigan Press, 1981: $12.50	Assessment manual Test booklet Stimulation activities	Handicapped children 0–36 months developmentally	Professionals	Assessment Programming Evaluation	Developmental Maturationist/ interactionist	Perceptual/Fine motor Cognition Language Social Self-Care Gross motor

Table 7.1: Continued

TEST	COMPONENTS	POPULATION AGE RANGE	USERS	PURPOSES	THEORETICAL FRAMEWORK	DOMAINS
B) Preschool Developmental Profile D.B. D'Eugenio and M.S. Moersch (eds), Ann Arbor: University of Michigan Press, 1981: $12.50	Assessment manual Test booklet Picture cards	Handicapped children 3–6 years developmentally	Professionals	Assessment Programming Evaluation	Developmental Maturationist/ interactionist	Perceptual/Fine motor Cognition Language Social Self-Care Gross motor
10. Vineland Adaptive Behaviour Scales S.S. Sparrow, D.A. Balla, and D.V. Cicchetti, Circle Pines, MN: American Guidance Service, 1984: $60.00	Expanded form Survey form Classroom form Computer software Cassette training tape (English and Spanish versions)	Persons 0–18 years	Professionals	Diagnosis Assessment Programming Evaluation	Functional	Communication Daily living skills Socialization Motor skills Maladaptive behaviour

2. *The Evaluation and Programming System: For Infants and Young Children, Developmentally 1 Month to 3 Years: Assessment Level I* (EPS-I) (Bricker, Gentry, and Bailey, 1985) is a criterion-referenced assessment instrument developed for children functioning developmentally between one month and three years, with a chronological age not exceeding six years. The instrument has two main purposes: to provide specific information that can be used to develop individual educational programmes across six developmental areas, and to be used as a tool to assess programme effectiveness (Bailey and Bricker, 1986). Six curricular domains are included in the EPS-I: Fine Motor, Gross Motor, Self-Care, Cognitive, Social-Communication, and Social. Each domain is divided into a series of content areas (Strands) which represent functionally uniform groups of conceptually related behaviours (e.g. problem-solving, prelinguistic communicative interactions, balance in sitting), meaning that the essential function or form of behaviours is the same throughout the strand. The EPS-I includes six recording forms containing the list of items for each domain and a supplementary social-communication recording form. A list of educational objectives is provided for each assessment item, and general guidelines are given for the development of IEP goals. A parallel form for parents to assess their children is included.

3. *The Brigance Diagnostic Inventory of Early Development* (Brigance, 1978) is a criterion-referenced instrument for children whose developmental level ranges from birth to 6 years and covers Psycho-Motor, Self-Help, Speech and Language, General Knowledge and Comprehension, and Early Academic Skills. In addition to the assessment component, educational objectives are provided for each assessment item, with general guidelines for the formulation of Individualized Education Program (IEP) goals.

4. *The Clinical and Educational Manual for Use with the Uzgiris and Hunt Scales of Infant Development* (Dunst, 1980) is designed to provide an overall profile and an Estimated Developmental Age (EDA) of a child's sensorimotor development between birth and 18 months of age, in addition to the stage placement as determined from the Ordinal Scales of Psychological Development (Uzgiris and Hunt, 1975). General guidelines are sug-

gested for the development of 'intervention packages'. More extensive suggestions of activities to teach 'critical behaviours' as measured in the assessment instrument are contained in a separate curriculum: *Infant Learning: A Cognitive-Linguistic Intervention Strategy* (Dunst, 1981).

5. The revised version of the *Hawaii Early Learning Profile* (HELP) (Furuno *et al.*, 1985) is a criterion-referenced assessment instrument and curriculum for young children aged from birth to three years of age. Over 650 items cover six developmental areas: Cognitive, Language, Fine Motor, Gross Motor, Social-Emotional, and Self-Help. The HELP consists primarily of an extensive activity guide which contains suggestions of activities and materials for specific skills. The assessment component includes a checklist and a profile chart.

6. *The Carolina Curriculum for Handicapped Infants and Infants At-Risk* (Johnson-Martin, Jens, and Attermeier, 1986) is designed primarily to provide curricular intervention strategies for children functioning developmentally between birth and 24 months. A checklist of 344 items is organized into six domains: Cognition, Communication/Language, Social Skills/Adaptation, Self-Help, Fine Motor and Gross Motor. Activities, materials, teaching procedures and programming steps are suggested for each item on the checklist.

7. *The Arizona Basic Assessment and Curriculum Utilization System* (ABACUS) (McCarthy, Lund, and Bos, 1986) is a comprehensive, criterion-referenced assessment, programming and evaluation system designed for children aged from two to five and a half years. Two hundred and fourteen items cover five domains: Body Management, Self-Care, Communication, Pre-Academics and Socialization. The ABACUS includes a screening scale, an assessment instrument, a programming component, an evaluation system for monitoring child progress, procedures for parent involvement and home teaching, and a programme supervision and evaluation system.

8. *The Battelle Developmental Inventory* (Newborg, Stock, Wnek, Guidubaldi, and Svinicki, 1984) is a standardized assessment battery for children aged from birth to eight years of age. It contains a screening component, and an assessment inventory of 341 items which covers five domains: Personal-Social,

Adaptive, Motor, Communication, and Cognitive. General procedures are provided for the formulation of educational objectives directly from the assessment item.

9. *Developmental Programming for Infants and Young Children* consists of two parts: a revised version of the Early Intervention Developmental Programming and Profile (EIDP) (Shafer and Moersch, 1981) and the Preschool Developmental Profile (PDP) (D'Eugenio & Moersch, 1981). The EIDP contains 299 items and was designed for children functioning developmentally between birth and 36 months; the PDP contains 213 items appropriate for older children functioning developmentally between three and six years of age. Both instruments are composed of six scales which provide developmental milestones in Perceptual/Fine Motor, Cognitive, Language, Social-Emotional, Self-Care, and Gross Motor development. The EIPD also provides a list of short term educational goals with suggested stimulation activities for each goal.

10. *The Vineland Adaptive Behaviour Scales* (Sparrow, Balla, and Cichetti, 1984), a revised version of the Vineland Social Maturity Scale (Doll, 1965), is a standardized instrument designed to assess adaptive behaviour in persons aged from birth to 18 years of age. The test is composed of three forms differing in length and purpose; the Expanded, the Survey and the Classroom Forms. Each form covers five domains: Communication, Daily Living Skills, Socialization, Motor Skills and Maladaptive Behaviours. General guidelines are given for the formulation of educational goals. The scale has both an English and a Spanish version.

The instruments described above can be considered curriculum-based assessments as they all address the issue of generating assessment information of relevance to instructional programming. Differences exist, however, in the focus of the assessment instruments and in the degree of specificity of curricular information. Most instruments (e.g. the Brigance, the Battelle, the Vineland) focus on the assessment component and provide only general guidelines for curricular programming. Others, such as the HELP and the Carolina concentrate primarily on curricula. Guidelines for evaluation procedures consist generally of suggestions for measuring child progress by pre and post intervention comparison of global test scores or of item-by-item progress.

Most of these assessment-curriculum systems have comprehensive content coverage, and include five to six developmental domains. The Clinical and Educational Manual focusses only on the Sensorimotor Cognitive domain. The age gap between skills varies among the instruments, depending on the total number of skills and the age range for which the test is designed.

Most assessments can be administered both in the classroom and in the home, and information is obtained from observation, direct test and by report. Except for the Portage and the Brigance, the scoring criteria allow for identification of inconsistent performance or emerging skills and the use of qualifying notes and comments, in addition to the mastery or failure of an item. A child's overall performance on a test is most often translated into an age level or a profile.

Table 2 provides a comparison of selected characteristics of the ten assessment-curriculum system including: 1) number of items, 2) type of items, 3) organization of items within domains, 4) type of adaptations specified for handicapping condition, 5) administration time, 6) data collection methods, 7) scoring options, 8) type of results, 9) standardization if applicable, and 10) psychometric data on the assessment and/or curriculum.

The remainder of this section compares and contrasts the ten assessment-curriculum systems in the following areas: theoretical framework, comprehensiveness, functionality, generality, instructional content, measurability, hierarchical relationships, psychometric data, and the linkage between the assessment and curricular components.

Table 7.2: Comparison of selected characteristics of reviewed assessment-curriculum systems (continued)

TEST	# OF ITEMS	TYPE OF ITEM	ORGANIZATION OF ITEMS WITHIN DOMAINS	ADAPTATIONS FOR HANDICAPS	ADMINISTRATION TIME	DATA COLLECTION METHODS	SCORING OPTIONS	TYPE OF RESULTS	STANDARD-IZATION	PSYCHOMETRIC DATA
1. The Portage 580 Guide to Early Education	580	Specific	Unrelated items sequenced according to age levels	None specified	None specified	Direct test	Pass	Age level	None	None
2. Evaluation and Programming System (EPS-1)	228	Generic	Developmental sequence related behaviours within strands	General guidelines for visual, motor and hearing impairments	1–2 hours	Observation Direct test Report	Pass Fail Inconsistent Qualifying notes Comments	Raw scores Percentages	None	Validity concurrent with Gesell (N=211) and Bailey (N=34) Reliability Interobserver (N=122) Test-Retest(N=55)

Table 7.2: Continued

TEST	# OF ITEMS	TYPE OF ITEM	ORGANIZATION OF ITEMS WITHIN DOMAINS	ADAPTATIONS FOR HANDICAPS	ADMINISTRATION TIME	DATA COLLECTION METHODS	SCORING OPTIONS	TYPE OF RESULTS	STANDARD-IZATION	PSYCHOMETRIC DATA
3. Brigance Diagnostic Inventory of Early Development	98 Skill sequences	Specific	Items sequenced according to age levels within general skill areas	General guidelines	Varies according to age	Observation Direct test Report	Pass Fail	Age level	None	None
4A. A Clinical and Educational Manual for Use with the Uzgiris and Hunt Scales of Infant Development	126	Generic	Developmental sequence of critical behaviours with substages	None specified	Not given	Observation Direct test	Pass Fail Inconsistent Qualifying notes Comments	Substage placement Developmental age Profile Deviation scores	na	Validity concurrent with Uzgiris and Hunt Scales and Griffith Reliability (Uzgiris and Hunt Scales) Interobserver Test-Retest

Table 7.2: Continued

TEST	# OF ITEMS	TYPE OF ITEM	ORGANIZATION OF ITEMS WITHIN DOMAINS	ADAPTATIONS FOR HANDICAPS	ADMINISTRATION TIME	DATA COLLECTION METHODS	SCORING OPTIONS	TYPE OF RESULTS	STANDARD-IZATION	PSYCHOMETRIC DATA
4B. Infant Learning: A Cognitive-Linguistic Intervention Strategy	na	na	na	na	na	na	na	na	na	na
5. Hawaii Early Learning Profile (HELP)	658	Specific Generic	Unrelated items sequenced according to age level	General guidelines for physical, auditory and visual impairments	None specified	Observation Direct test Report	Pass Fail Emerging Report Comments	Pass Fail Emerging Report Comments	None	None

Table 7.2: Continued

TEST	# OF ITEMS	TYPE OF ITEM	ORGANIZATION OF ITEMS WITHIN DOMAINS	ADAPTATIONS FOR HANDICAPS	ADMINISTRATION TIME	DATA COLLECTION METHODS	SCORING OPTIONS	TYPE OF RESULTS	STANDARD-IZATION	PSYCHOMETRIC DATA
6. The Carolina Curriculum for Handicapped Infants and Infants at Risk	344	Specific Generic	Developmental sequence items within areas of related behaviours	Specific adaptations for visual and motor impairments	None specified	Observation Direct test Report	Pass Emerging	Pass Emerging	None	None
7. Arizona Basic Assessment and Curriculum for Young Children with Special Needs (ABACUS)	214	Specific	Developmental sequence of items within subareas	None specified	None specified	Direct test	Pass Fail	Pass Fail	None	None

Table 7.2: Continued

TEST	# OF ITEMS	TYPE OF ITEM	ORGANIZATION OF ITEMS WITHIN DOMAINS	ADAPTATIONS FOR HANDICAPS	ADMINISTRATION TIME	DATA COLLECTION METHODS	SCORING OPTIONS	TYPE OF RESULTS	STANDARD-IZATION	PSYCHOMETRIC DATA
8. Battelle Developmental Inventory	341	Specific	Items grouped by age ranges within subdomains	General guidelines for motor visual and hearing impairments and emotional disability	1.5-2 hours	Observation Direct test Report	Typically Sometimes Never Comments	Age level Standard scores	Normal population (N= 800)	Validity Content (expert) Construct (factorial validity) Criterion (Vineland, DASI, Stanford-Binet, WISC-R, PPVT) Reliability Interrater (N=143) Test-Retest (N=183) Standard Error

Table 7.2: Continued

TEST	# OF ITEMS	TYPE OF ITEM	ORGANIZATION OF ITEMS WITHIN DOMAINS	ADAPTATIONS FOR HANDICAPS	ADMINISTRATION TIME	DATA COLLECTION METHODS	SCORING OPTIONS	TYPE OF RESULTS	STANDARD-IZATION	PSYCHOMETRIC DATA
9. Developmental Programming for Infants and Young Children A) Early Intervention Developmental Programming and Profile (Revised version)	299	Specific Generic	Unrelated items grouped within age ranges	General guidelines	1 hour	Direct test	Pass Fail Inconsistent Omitted	Age level Profile	None	Validity Content (expert review) Concurrent (N=14 handicapped children) Consistency of performance across scales(N=14) Reliability Interobserver (100 items) Test-Retest(N=15)

Table 7.2: Continued

TEST	# OF ITEMS	TYPE OF ITEM	ORGANIZATION OF ITEMS WITHIN DOMAINS	ADAPTATIONS FOR HANDICAPS	ADMINISTRATION TIME	DATA COLLECTION METHODS	SCORING OPTIONS	TYPE OF RESULTS	STANDARD-IZATION	PSYCHOMETRIC DATA
B) Preschool Developmental Profile	213	Specific Generic	Unrelated items grouped within age ranges	None specified	1 hour	Direct test	Pass Fail Inconsistent Omitted	Age level Profile	None	Validity Content Reliability Cognitive scale only: Interobserver Scalogram

Table 7.2: Continued

TEST	# OF ITEMS	TYPE OF ITEM	ORGANIZATION OF ITEMS WITHIN DOMAINS	ADAPTATIONS FOR HANDICAPS	ADMINISTRATION TIME	DATA COLLECTION METHODS	SCORING OPTIONS	TYPE OF RESULTS	STANDARD-IZATION	PSYCHOMETRIC DATA
10. Vineland Adaptive Behaviour Scales	577	Specific	Developmental sequence of items within subdomains	None specified	20–90 minutes	Observation Direct test Report	Usually Sometimes Never No opportunity Don't know	Age levels Maladaptive level Standard scores	Normal population (N= 3000)	Validity Construct: developmental progression, factor analysis Content criterion: with other adaptive behaviour scales, Kaufman, PPVT Reliability Internal consistency Test-Retest (N=484) Interrater (N=160)

COMPARISON OF ASSESSMENT-CURRICULUM SYSTEMS

Theoretical Framework

Because models of development yield different implications for assessment and intervention, consideration should be given to the theoretical framework underlying the development of the assessment instruments and the curricula. A maturationist perspective, for example, emphasizes the description of developmental milestones dependent on internal maturation processes, the establishment of norms, and an experiential, non-structured approach to teaching (Dunst, 1981). A behavioural approach focuses on the identification of task-related behaviours (specific skills), the use of arbitrarily set criteria for measuring performance (Fewell, 1983), and a programmed learning, teacher-directed orientation to teaching (Bailey, Jens, and Johnson, 1983). An interactional/transactional framework takes into account both the developmental characteristics of the child's functioning behaviours, and skills are taught as they occur within daily activities (Dunst, 1981).

Most of the systems reviewed base their content on a developmental maturationist framework, as most items were selected from traditional standardized tests. The Portage contains many items taken from the Bayley; the Carolina contains items derived from developmental skills listed on the Bayley, the Gesell, and the Cattell; the Brigance contains items from the Bayley, the Gesell, the Griffiths, and the Stanford-Binet. The EIDP and the PDP developed items from a review of the literature of Piagetian theory, studies on infant cognition, attachment and acquisition of ego theories, and neurodevelopmental theories of reflexive development. The content covered in the Clinical and Educational Manual and the Infant Learning Curriculum is based primarily on the Neo-Piagetian literature and research. The content in the EPS-I is based on a developmental-functional approach. Conditions for inclusion of items in the EPS-I were that skills were considered functional, generic, and thus easy to embed within daily activities. Items are organized according to developmental and logical teaching sequences. The ABACUS is based on an ecological approach, and covers important developmental skills which are also functional behaviours for children within their social and physical environment.

Some instruments are eclectic in their adherence to a theoretical framework. While most items contained in the Battelle, for example, are derived from a developmental milestones approach, the instructional strategies proposed are typically behavioural. Similarly, the ABACUS prescribes direct instruction teaching strategies, despite the stated ecological orientation of the system. The Clinical and Educational Manual, combined with the Infant Learning curriculum is a fine example of theoretical consistency within a developmental-interactionist-ecological approach, linking Piagetian-based content to activity-based instructional strategies.

Comprehensiveness

The assessment of young children with special needs requires instruments that are comprehensive in nature (Simeonssen, Huntington, and Parse, 1980). The behaviours of infants and young children are only arbitrarily categorized into domains of development. In reality, the overlap between some domains is so substantial that there is little consistency in organization across test instruments. For example, of the tests reviewed, similar skills are contained in domains labelled Fine Motor, Cognitive, Pre-Academics, Perceptual/Fine Motor, and Early Academics: fitting pieces into puzzles, stacking, releasing small objects into containers.

One of the most valuable aspects of programmatic assessment is the provision of a baseline from which to develop and monitor subsequent instructional goals and objectives (Bagnato and Neisworth, 1981). The development of a comprehensive educational plan necessitates a comprehensive assessment across all major domains of development, over time and across settings.

Most of the instruments reviewed include all domains in a single instrument The Clinical and Educational Manual and the Infant Learning Curriculum are notable exceptions, addressing specific 'critical' Piagetian-based cognitive behaviours in depth.

Functionality

The usefulness of a skill in increasing a child's ability to interact within the daily environment is a major factor for determining the utility of assessment items to serve as a basis for the formulation of educational goals. Many items derived from traditional standardized tests consist of skills too specific to be of relevance to everyday functioning. Teaching a child to place pegs in a pegboard is less conducive to improving the child's coping within the daily environment than teaching the use of pincer grasp to pick up small objects, such as buttons, raisins or cereals. In addition, items derived from standardized tests refer to skills and materials which are, for the most part, specific to Western cultures, and therefore may hold little if any, functional relevance within non-Western oriented systems.

Another problem with the derivation of items from instruments based on developmental milestone framework is that skills that differentiate children by age are not always critical skills to teach (Bailey, Jens, and Johnson, 1983). Some of the tests reviewed were found to contain items of questionable desirability for the child to learn, such as 'Walked backward, toe to heel six steps' (Brigance), 'Talks in loud urgent voice' (HELP), or 'Runs stiffly' (Carolina), as compared to more generic exploratory, dressing and feeding skills. The EPS-I contains primarily functional skills. In the Fine Motor Domain, for example, Strand B: Functional Use of Fine Motor Skills contains items such as 'Fits objects into a defined space', and 'Uses either hand to activate an object'.

Generality

Because of the nature and purpose of standardized tests, the items included are usually situation, material and person specific. Such specificity is of questionable utility in providing information on the child's actual functioning within the daily environment, across settings, materials and people (Johnson, 1982). The assessment and teaching of skills, such as 'Places raisins in a bottle' (Battelle), , and 'Imitates building a two-block tower' (Carolina) do not give a representative picture of a child's actual functioning, nor do they examine generalization across materials and settings. Also such items do not allow for adaptations. More generic behaviours, such as 'Imitates simple, familiar gestures', 'Places object into a container', 'Initiates and maintains communictive exchange with familiar adult' (EPS-I) focus on underlying concepts which can be operationally defined in different manners and easily adapted to suit the idiosyncrasies in response capabilities of atypical children (Robinson and Robinson, 1983).

The emphasis on function and process, rather than on form and product, is of relevance for the assessment of cognitive and social-communication skills of children with sensory-impairements. Because items in traditional infant measures largely tap sensory and motor capacities, they do not accurately reflect the infant's cognitive and communication competence (Bornstein and Sigman, 1986; Vietze and Coates, 1986). Items such as 'Pulls open drawers and cupboard doors' (Battelle), 'Looks for object that has disappeared' (ABACUS), 'Identifies self in mirror' (Battelle) are too restrictive, and exclude the variety of alternative ways a child who has visual or motor impairment might use to explore the environment, locate objects, and demonstrate identity of self. Most of the tests mention the importance of modifying items for sensory impairments, but many items included in most of the tests are mode and situation specific. In the Brigance, the EIDP, the PDP, and the Battelle, the adaptations recommended are general logical guidelines. Only the Carolina and the EPS-I contain adequate information, either by emphasizing generic skills such as 'Persists in effort to obtain something' (Carolina), 'Participates in game' (Carolina), 'Uses an object to obtain another object' (EPS-I), 'Gains attention and refers to object, person, and/or event' (EPS-I) or by providing alternative items like those suggested for assessing object permanence in visually impaired children such as, 'Reaches for object after it no longer makes a noise' (Carolina).

Cross cultural studies (e.g. Greenfield, 1976) illustrate the importance of taking into consideration the cultural specificity of tasks and materials when studying development within non-Western oriented systems. For example, non-Western populations do not necessarily perform in a manner similar to Western-oriented populations on Piagetian developmental tasks, unless presented with tasks and materials which are familiar and appropriate to their culture (Fischer and Silvern, 1985). Assessment and curriculum systems which focus on generic underlying concepts and processes allow for the identification of specific, representative behaviours and the use of tasks and materials which are familiar and appropriate to the child's particular cultural environment.

Instructional Context

An underlying premise which seems to have been overlooked in the development of most assessment-curriculum systems is that the characteristics of items differ according to the purpose for which the test is designed. Items included in diagnostic tools are chosen for their ability to describe normative development and to discriminate the behaviours of children at different ages. Assessment tools designed for programming purposes focus on the identification of skills that are functional for an individual child and that can be taught within the child's daily environment. The indiscriminate inclusion of developmental milestones in programmatic assessment instruments fails to acknowledge that a skill's diagnostic and developmental importance does not necessarily imply the same skill's functionality or educational relevance. Many skills considered to be developmental milestones cannot be taught, such as the following example taken from the Brigance: 'Stops crying in anticipation of care or attention when someone enters the room, while not experiencing genuine discomfort'.

Items restricted to specific materials and settings do not lend themselves to the formulation of educational goals which can be easily integrated by teachers and parents within daily routines. The teaching of such skills often requires implementation out of context in a manner that does not reflect the way the child will use the skill in the daily environment and limits the opportunities for the child to generalize a newly taught skill (Johnson, 1982). To focus on teaching a child to place raisins in a bottle, for example, ignores the many other opportunities the child may have to place small objects in containers.

The content of an item also yields implications for the selection of teaching strategies. Specificity of materials and settings usually requires that special circumstances be set up to elicit targeted responses, as opposed to an activity-based instructional approach which allows young children to engage in activities of interest. Few of the tests reviewed specifically delineate teaching procedures within an activity-based framework, despite stated adherence to functional and ecological orientations. Some items and teaching procedures in the Battelle and the ABACUS, for example, lack the generalizability necessary for easy integration within daily activities. Items included in the EPS-I reflect conceptual or response classes (e.g. 'stacks objects', 'entertains self by playing appropriately with toys', 'jumps from low platform'), rather than singular, specific responses. These items allow for modifications and easy integration within daily activities across a variety of materials and settings. The Clinical and Educational Manual and the Infant Learning curriculum specify procedures and examples of how to embed targeted skills (e.g. obtaining completely hidden objects) within functional daily activities (e.g. looking for objects placed in drawers, cupboards, sand, bubblebath, palm of hand, handbag), as compared to the traditional procedures of hiding objects under a piece of cloth or behind a screen.

Measurability

For reliability and evaluation purposes, skills need to be observable, measurable and contain specific criteria for mastery. Items such as 'Expresses enthusiasm for work and play' (Battelle), 'Asserts self in acceptable way' (Battelle), or 'Tries to please others' (Carolina), for example, require inferences by the test administrator. The lack of operational criteria may result in differential interpretations between observers or by the same observer across times. Criteria for mastery of a skill are lacking in the checklists of the Portage, the HELP, the Carolina, and, in part, the Brigance. The Portage and the Carolina, however, specify criteria in their curriculum component. Items in the EPS-I are worded in observable and measurable terms and specific criteria for mastery are indicated.

Hierarchical Relationship

A hierarchical, sequential organization of items within groups of related behaviours (e.g. causality, transition to words, balance and mobility in standing and walking) enables the identification of skill the child is ready to learn next. The skill sequence provides the interventionist with a consistent training progression of conceptually related subskills within a generic class of behaviours, and serves as a reference for the identification of IEP annual goals and short-term objectives.

The typical ordering of items in standardized diagnostic tests, according to mean ages at which the skill is observed in normal children, usually results in sequences of relatively unrelated behaviours. The sequence of the items is meant to emphasize age discrimination, rather than continuity in the development of a skill over time. The organization of the items in most of the systems reviewed lacks the continuity necessary to provide a logical teaching sequence in which a recently learned skill can be practised as a more difficult skill is taught.

The Cognitive domain of the HELP, for example, contains sequences such as 'Distinguishes between friendly and angry voices', 'Points to distant objects outdoors', 'Pastes on appropriate side'. The Portage is organized in a similar manner, containing sequences such as, in the Self-help domain, 'Helps mother when drying hands and face', 'Indicates when wet or soiled', 'Puts hat on head and takes it off'. Similar sequences of unrelated behaviours are found in the Brigance, the EIDP, and the Battelle.

In the Carolina the basis for the sequencing of items seems to vary. A logical teaching sequence for developing functional use of objects in symbolic play is reflected in a progression of items such as 'Moves hand to mouth', 'Explores objects with mouth', 'Plays with (e.g., shakes or bangs) toys placed in hand'. The teaching logic of the sequence is less evident in other areas as, for example, in the sequence 'Responds differently to strangers versus familiar people', 'Participates in games', 'Repeats activity that is laughed at', contained in the social skills area. The organization of test items in the ABACUS also lacks a consistent hierarchical teaching sequence, but the curriculum component provides a breakdown of each item into logical teaching steps.

In contrast, items in the Clinical and Educational Manual are, for the most part, organized in sequences such as 'Uses some form of locomotion as a means to obtain an out of reach object', 'Pushes obstruction (e.g., pillow or Plexiglass) out of the way to obtain an object', 'Pulls support to obtain an object placed on it', which represents a logical teaching progression within the area of the development of means for obtaining desired environmental effects.

Test items in the EPS-I are also organized according to a developmental and logical teaching sequence. Each domain is divided into a series of strands. Each strand contains a series of items called Long Range Goals (LRG) and Training Objectives (TO), more discrete skills arranged in a developmental and/or hierarchical training progression, which enable the pinpointing of the child's level within a specific sequence.

Psychometric Information

Only two of the tests reviewed, the Battelle and the Vineland, have been normed and provide standard scores. The standardization samples (N = 800 and N = 3000, respectively) are small, however, when broken down into individual age groups. Neither test presents adequate information on the representation of populations with handicaps in standardization samples. The Clinical and Educational Manual gives deviation scores to identify the existence and extent of a developmental delay. The scores were determined clinically as opposed to empirically.

Similarly, the age levels indicated in the remaining systems that report them, lack empirical bases. The assignment of items to ages, such as in the EIDP, is taken from standardization data collected on a variety of other assessment instruments (e.g. Gesell, Bayley). Some tests combine published norms across multiple references (e.g. the Brigance, the HELP), resulting in age levels with such wide ranges as to be of questionable use for young populations. For example, some items in the HELP can be passed within a six month age range. 'Scribbles spontaneously', for example, can be passed between 13 and 18 months; 'Explores cabinet and drawers', between 18 and 24 months.

Except for the Battelle and the Vineland, psychometric data on the validity and reliability of the criterion-referenced tests are lacking, and when given, the sample sizes are small.

The EPS-I is the exception, as relatively extensive data have been collected on the assessment portion of this system (Bricker, 1988). Interobserver reliability ranged from 0.70 on the social domain to 0.95 on the gross motor domain, and 0 .87 (*N*=122) for the total test. Test-retest reliability ranged from 0.77 for the social domain to 0.95 for the gross motor domain with a mean agreement of 0.87 (*N*=55). In terms of validity, correlations between children's performance on the EPS-I and the Gesell (*N*=121) was 0.509 (*p* less than 0.001), 0.88 for the psycho-motor scale, and 0.93 for the mental scale of the Bayley (*N*=34) (*p* less than 0.001). These data were collected for children who ranged in age from two months to six years, and included non-handicapped, at-risk, mild, moderate and severely handicapped children. Analysis of the internal consistency of the EPS-I was examined by correlating strand scores to domain scores and domain scores to total scores (*N*=155). The correlations for strand to domain ranged from 0.60 to 0.95 indicating substantial relationships between strands and domains. The correlations for domains to total test ranged from 0.89 to 0.98.

The utility of the EPS-I for programming was also investigated in a well-controlled study involving 48 early interventionists from 3 States and British Columbia (Notari, 1988).

The experimental groups that used the EPS-I wrote significantly better LRGs and STOs. In particular, the EPS-I provided guidance in the identification of specific long term expectations for children, which were developmentally and educationally consistent with the STOs.

No empirical research is reported for any of the curriculum components, except for a first version of the Carolina. For editions published in the United States, no information is available on the standardization or on the utility of any of the assessment-curriculum systems for populations outside of North America.

Linkage Between Assessment and Curriculum

The most common and economical way to link assessment and curriculum is to make test items identical to curriculum goals. The items which are assessed are also the skills that are selected as educational targets. The skill chosen as an educational goal is usually the assessment item which immediately follows the most developmentally advanced of the skills mastered by the child.

The systems reviewed present notable differences in the degree to which they offer specific programming information. Some of the instruments (i.e. Brigance, Battelle, Vineland) focus primarily on assessment and contain only general guidelines on procedures for formulating educational goals directly from the test items. The Battelle, for example, suggests that the test administration materials and criteria be used as teaching procedures, materials and criteria for mastery. The EPS-I contains a list of objectives for each assessment item, as well as general guidelines for the development of IEP goals. The Brigance provides standard phrases for the wording of IEP goals with blanks to complete by writing the targeted objective. The Portage, EIDP, HELP, Infant Learning, and Carolina offer curriculum guides containing suggestions for activities and teaching procedures for all or part of the assessment items. The ABACUS curriculum also contains additional skills not measured in the assessment component. All of the assessment items are cross-referenced in the curriculum, but assessment and curriculum components differ in the sequence and grouping of the skills, because assessment items are not sequenced according to a logical teaching progression.

Table 3 presents the methods each of the ten assessment-curriculum systems uses for linking their assessment and curricular components and provides a comparison of the curricular content, instructional strategies, adaptations, and measures of child progress for the systems. All of the curriculum guides reviewed (Portage, EIDP, HELP, Infant Learning, Carolina, ABACUS) contain a variety of excellent suggestions of activities and materials for each educational goal.

Table 7.3: Comparison of methods for linking assessment-curriculum components, curriculum content, instructional strategies, adaptations and measures of child progress for reviewed assessment-curriculum systems

TEST	METHOD FOR LINKING ASSESSMENT AND CURRICULUM	CURRICULUM CONTENT	INSTRUCTIONAL STRATEGIES	CURRICULUM ADAPTATIONS	MEASURES OF CHILD PROGRESS
1. The Portage Guide to Early Education	Specific activities are suggested for each test item	Activities Materials Criteria for mastery	Behavioural	None specified	Item by item Age level
2. Evaluation and Programming System (EPS-1)	Objectives are listed for each test item Test items linked to curricular activities and programming steps	Importance of skill Activities Materials Teaching procedures Programming steps	Behavioural-activity-based	Specific consideration for visual, motor and hearing impairment	Item by item Test scores
3. Brigance Diagnostic Inventory of Early Development	Objectives are listed for each test item	None specified	None specified	None specified	Item by item Age level

Table 7.3: Continued

TEST	METHOD FOR LINKING ASSESSMENT AND CURRICULUM	CURRICULUM CONTENT	INSTRUCTIONAL STRATEGIES	CURRICULUM ADAPTATIONS	MEASURES OF CHILD PROGESS
4A. A Clinical and Educational Manual for Use with the Uzgiris and Hunt Scales of Infant Development	General guidelines for the development of 'intervention packages' with examples (case studies)	None specified	None specified	None specified	None specified
4B. Infant Learning: A Cognitive-Linguistic Intervention Strategy	Specific activities are suggested for critical behaviours measured in Piagetian assessments	Explanation of skills Materials Activities	Activity-based	None specified	None specified
5. Hawaii Early Leaning Profile (HELP)	General guidelines for formulating objectives Specific activities are suggested for each test item	Explanation of skills Materials Activities	Experiential Activity-based	None specified	Item by item Charting change

Table 7.3: Continued

TEST	METHOD FOR LINKING ASSESSMENT AND CURRICULUM	CURRICULUM CONTENT	INSTRUCTIONAL STRATEGIES	CURRICULUM ADAPTATIONS	MEASURES OF CHILD PROGESS
6. The Carolina Curriculum for Handicapped Infants and Infants at Risk	General guidelines for writing educational goals Activities suggested for each test item	Activities Materials Teaching procedures Programming steps	Behavioural activity-based	Specific suggestions for visual, motor and hearing impairments	Item by item
7. Arizona Basic Assessment and Curriculum for Young Children with Special Needs (ABACUS)	Each item is cross-referenced with a task and program in the curriculum Guidelines for writing goals	Activities Materials Teaching procedures Programming steps	Behavioural	General guidelines	Item by item Guidelines for monitoring progress and programming decision-making
8. Battelle Developmental Inventory	General guidelines for developing objectives for each test item	None specified	None specified	None specified	Item by item Standard score

Table 7.3: Continued

TEST	METHOD FOR LINKING ASSESSMENT AND CURRICULUM	CURRICULUM CONTENT	INSTRUCTIONAL STRATEGIES	CURRICULUM ADAPTATIONS	MEASURES OF CHILD PROGESS
9. Developmental Programming for Infants and Young Children A) Early Intervention Developmental Programming and Profile (Revised version)	General guidelines for formulating goals Short term goals with specific activities are provided for each developmental age range	Activities Materials	Behavioural Activity-based	Specific adaptations for hearing, motorically and visually impaired children	Item by item Age range
B) Preschool Developmental Profile	None specified	None specified	None specified	None specified	Item by item Age range
10. Vineland Adaptive Behaviour Scales	General guidelines for formulating goals from test items	None specified	None specified	None specified	Test scores

Only the EIDP activity guide and the Carolina mention specific item adaptations for motor and sensory impairments. In the Carolina, for teaching spatial concepts (e.g. 'Puts objects away in correct places') to a physically disabled child, it is suggested that the teacher put away an object and then ask the child whether the location was correct. The other curricula only contain general guidelines for adaptations.

Instructional strategies vary from ecological, activity-based approaches (Infant Learning) to specific suggestions of instructional cues and prompts to train detailed skills, and task analysed into smaller components (e.g. ABACUS). Many curricula (e.g. the Carolina) allow for the use of different strategies, proposing experiential learning approaches, and including additional suggestions of instructional cues and prompts if needed.

Eight of the assessment-curriculum systems suggest measures of child progress, such as number of items successfully completed by children, monitoring change in age level, test scores and standard scores.

CONCLUSION

The assessment-curriculum systems reviewed each have specific advantages and disadvantages. The instruments are comprehensive as to their content, which, in general, draws largely from traditional developmental milestones, although some tests (i.e. EIDP, Carolina) have included information from more recent literature and research. Problems still remain as to the educational relevance of the items derived from a developmental milestone framework, as skills that differentiate children by age are not always critical to children's independent functioning. Their specificity, due to standardization requirements, limits the extent and relevance of the information on the child's functioning within the daily environment and ignores the many opportunities the child might have to learn and practise a skill over a variety of settings and materials.

An inconsistency among items as to the functionality of their content, as well as a lack of organization of skills according to a logical teaching sequence was found in most of the assessment instruments. This raises some concern about the relevance of the assessment information, when used for programming purposes, especially if the test only provides general guidelines for rewording assessment items into education goals. The curricula reviewed generally contain excellent suggestions for activities. As in the assessment components, however, skills are usually not organized into groups of related behaviours nor sequenced according to a developmental and logical teaching progression.

Most of the criterion-referenced instruments lack empirical support for assigning age levels. Age levels are based on norms for individual items selected from a variety of existing standardized tests. The utilization of only selected items in new tests invalidates norms, as norms for most tests are computed on an overall basis, rather than on an item basis (Sheehan, 1982).

A major concern also expressed by Bailey, Jens, and Johnson (1983), and Sheehan (1982) is the overall lack of adequate reliability and validity data. Among the instruments reviewed, only the Battelle, the Vineland and the EPS-I have extensive data on their reliability and validity.

Also, all of the instruments were devised within a Western cultural context. No information is available on their use outside of a Western society. Of the instruments reviewed, those which focus on skills representing generic underlying concepts would seem to present an advantage for identifying skills and using materials of functional relevance to non-Western oriented cultures.

Although problems still exist with available assessment-curriculum systems, most tests specifically mention programming as a primary purpose, and attempt to provide guidelines for linking assessment and curriculum. The use of these assessment-curriculum systems can greatly assist early intervention personnel in linking assessment and intervention content for several reasons. First, the assessment component for most systems provides a systematic and comprehensive picture of a child's daily functioning. Clearly some instruments provide superior information, but almost all provide objective information on important skills children can and cannot perform.

Second, most systems have general or specific procedures to permit effective formulation of IEP long-range goals and short-term objectives based on the assessment information. Third, many systems contain associated curricula either of a specific or general nature. The delineation of specific curricular content and materials can be of enormous use to interventionists in designing functional and generic lessons plans.

Fourth, some of the systems are designed so that skills are arranged into meaningful, relevant goals and objectives that are hierarchically arranged. Such hierarchical arrangements assist parents and interventionists in appreciating logical sequences of development and in planning intervention targets that take into account such developmental progressions.

Finally, most systems provide the user with concrete strategies for monitoring children's change over time. The presence of evaluation procedures suggests to interventionists the necessity of evaluating intervention efforts as well as providing practical implementation strategies.

To summarize, we recommend that early interventionists take into consideration the following points in the selection of assessment and curriculum systems:

1. The systems should contain assessment, curriculum, and evaluation components.
2. Procedures for linking components should be direct and easy to implement.
3. Empirical data should be available on the psychometric qualities of the assessment component and on the educational relevance of the curriculum.
4. The curriculum should reflect developmentally important skills which are functional, generic, and can be meaningfully integrated in daily activities within a variety of cultural environments.
5. Guidelines should be provided for formulating educational programmes consisting of skills organized according to logical teaching sequence.
6. Evaluation procedures should enable easy and regular monitoring of child progress.

The field of early intervention has made significant progress since its inception in the early 1970s. We believe one of the most significant contributions has been the advent of linked assessment-curriculum systems. The refinement of these systems will be a major contribution of the 1990s.

REFERENCES

Apgar, V. (1953) 'A Proposal for a New Method of Evaluation of the Newborn Infant,' *Anesthesia and Analgesia, 32*, 260–267.

Bagnato, S.J. and Neisworth, J.T. (1981) *Linking Developmental Assessment and Curricula: Prescriptions for Early Intervention*, Aspen Systems, Rockville, MD.

Bagnato, S.J., Neisworth, J.T. and Capone, A. (1986) 'Curriculum-Based Assessment for the Young Exceptional Child: Rationale and Review,' *Topics in Early Childhood Special Education, 6*(2), 97–110.

Bailey, E.J. (1983) *Psychometric Evaluation of the Early Comprehensive Evaluation and Programming System*, unpublished doctoral dissertation, University of Oregon, Eugene, OR.

Bailey, E.J. and Bricker, D.D. (1986) 'A Psychometric Study of a Criterion-Referenced Assessment Instrument Designed for Infants and Young Children,' *Journal of the Division for Early Childhood, 10*(2), 124–134.

Bailey, E.J., Jens, K. and Johnson, N. (1983) 'Curricula for handicapped infants,' in S.G. Garwood and R.R. Fewell (eds), *Educating Handicapped Infants: Issues in Development and Intervention*, Rockville, Aspen, CO.

Bayley, N. (1969) *Bayley Scales of Infant Development*, The Psychological Corporation, Inc., New York.

Bereiter, C. and Englemann, S. (1966) *Teaching Disadvantaged Children in the Preschool*, Prentice-Hall, Englewood Cliffs, NJ.

Bluma, A., Shearer, M., Frohman, A. and Hilliard, J. (1976) *The Portage Guide to Early Education*, The Portage Project, CESA 12, Portage, WI.

Bornstein, M.H. and Sigman, M.D. (1986) 'Continuity in Mental Development from Infancy,' *Child Development, 57*(2), 251–274.

Bricker, D.D. (1986) *Early Education of At-Risk and Handicapped Infants, Toddlers, and Preschool Children*, Scott, Foresman and Company, Glenview, IL.

Bricker, D.D. (1988) Psychometric and Utility Study of a Comprehensive Early Assessment Instrument for Handicapped Infants and Children, final report for Grant G008400661 from the US Office of Education and Rehabilitative Services to Centre on Human Development, University of Oregon, Eugene, OR.

Bricker, D.D. (1989) *Early Intervention for At-Risk and Handicapped Infants, Toddlers, and Preschool Children*, Vort Corporation, Palo Alto, CA.

Bricker, D., Bailey, E., and Slentz, K. (in press) 'Reliability, Validity and Utility of the Evaluation and Programming System: For Infants and Young Children (EPS-I),' *Journal of Early Intervention*.

Bricker, D.D., Gentry, D. and Bailey, E.J. (1985) *Evaluation and Programming System: For Infants and Young Children: Assessment Level I: Developmentally 1 Month to 3 Years*, University of Oregon, Eugene, OR.

Bricker, D.D. and Littman, D. (1982) 'Intervention and Evaluation: The Inseparable Mix,' *Topics in Early Childhood Special Education*, 1, 23–33.

Brigance, A. (1978) *Inventory of Early Development*, Curriculum Associates, North Billerica, MA.

Bronfenbrenner, U. (1979) *The Ecology of Human Development: Experiments of Nature and Design*, Harvard University Press, Cambridge, MA.

D'Eugenio, D.B. and Moersch, M.S. (eds) (1981) *Preschool Developmental Profile*, University of Michigan Press, Ann Arbor, MI.

Doll, E.A. (1965) *Vineland Social Maturity Scale*, American Guidance Service, Circle Pines, Minnesota.

Dunst, C.J. (1980) *A Clinical and Educational Manual for Use with the Uzgiris and Hunt Scales of Infant Development*, University Park Press, Baltimore, MD

Dunst, C.J. (1981) *Infant Learning: A Cognitive-Linguistic Intervention Strategy*, DLM Teaching Resources, Allen, TX.

Dunst, C.J. (1986) 'Overview of the Efficacy of Early Intervention Programs,' in L. Bickman and D. Weatherford (eds), *Evaluating Early Intervention Programs ofr Severely Handicapped Children and Their Families*, Pro-Ed: Austin, TX.

Dunst, C.J. and Rheingrove, R. (1981) 'An Analysis of the Efficacy of Infant Intervention Programs with Organically Handicapped Children,' *Evaluation and Program Planning*, 4, 287–323.

Fewell, R. (1983) 'Assessing Handicapped Infants,' in G. Garwood and R. Fewell (eds), *Educating Handicapped Infants*, Aspen, Rockville, MD.

Fischer, K.W. and Silvern, L. (1985) 'Stages and individual differences in cognitive development,' *Annual Review of Psychology*, 36, 613–648.

Forman, G.E. and Hill, F. (1984) *Constructive Play: Applying Piaget in the Preschool*, Brooks/Cole, Monterey, CA.

Frankenburg, W., Dodds, J., Fandal, A., Kuzak, E. and Cohrs, M. (1975) *Denver Developmental Screening Test: Reference Manual (revised 1975 ed.)*, LADOCA Project and Publishing Foundation, Denver, CO.

Franklin, M.B. and Biber, B. (1977) 'Psychological Perspective and Early Childhood Education: Some Relations Between Theory and Practice,' in L.G. Katz (ed.), *Current Topics in Early Childhood Education (vol. 1)*, Ablex, Norwood, NJ.

Furuno, S., O'Reilly, K.A., Hosaka, C.M., Inatsuka, T.T., Allman T.L., and Zeisloft-Falbey, B (1985) *Hawaii Early Learning Profile (rev. ed)*, VORT, Palo Alto, CA.

Garwood, G. (1982) 'Early Childhood Intervention: Is It Time to Change Outcome Variables?,' *Topics in Early Childhood Special Education, 1*, ix–xi.

Greenfield, P.M. (1976) 'Cross Cultural Research and Piagetian Theory: Paradox and Progress,' in K.F. Riegel and J.A. Meacham (eds), *The Developing Individual in a Changing World, (Vol. 1)*, Mouton, The Hague.

Guess, D. and Siegel-Causey, E. (1983) 'Behavioral Control and Education of Severely Handicapped Students: Who's Doing What to Whom? and Why?,' in D. Bricker and J. Filler (eds), *Serving the Severely Retarded: From Research to Practice*, The Council for Exceptional Children, Reston, VA.

Hamilton, J. and Swan, W. (1981) 'Measurement References in the Assessment of Preschool Handicapped Children,' *Topics in Early Childhood Special Education, 1*(2), 42–48.

Hobbs, N. (1975) *The Futures of Children*, Jossey-Bass, San Francisco.

Hofmann, G., Banet, B. A., and Weikart, D. P. (1979) *Young Children in Action*, The High/Scope Press, Ypsilanti, Michigan.

Johnson, L. and Beauchamp, K. (1987) 'Preschool Assessment Measures: What are Teachers Using?,' *Journal of the Division for Early Childhood, 12*(1), 70–76.

Johnson, N. (1982) 'An Interventionist's Perspective,' in D. Bricker (ed), *Intervention with At-risk and Handicapped Infants: From Research to Application*, University Park Press, Baltimore.

Johnson-Martin, N., Jens, K. and Attermeier, S. (1986) *The Carolina Curriculum for Handicapped Infants and Infants At-Risk*, Paul H. Brookes, Baltimore.

Kamii, C. and DeVries, R. (1978) *Physical Knowledge in Preschool Education*, Prentice-Hall, Englewood Cliffs, NJ

McCarthy, J.M., Lund, K.A. and Bos, C.S. (1987) *The Arizona Basic Assessment and Curriculum Utilization System*, Love Publishing Co., Denver.

Newborg, J., Stock, J., Wnek, L., Guidubaldi, J. and Svinicki, J. (1984) *Battelle Developmental Inventory*, DLM Teaching Resources, Allen, TX.

Notari, A. (1988) *The Utility of a Criterion-Referenced Instrument in the Development of Individualized Education Plans for Infants and Young Children*, unpublished doctoral dissertation, University of Oregon, Eugene, OR.

Robinson, C.C. and Robinson, J.H. (1983) 'Sensorimotor Functions and Cognitive Development,' in M. Snell (ed.), *Systematic Instruction of the Moderately and Severely Handicapped* (2nd ed.), Charles E. Merrill, Columbus, OH.

Schwartz, S.L. and Robinson, H.F. (1982) *Designing Curriculum for Early Childhood*, Allyn and Bacon, Boston.

Shafer, D.S. and Moersch, M.S. (eds) (1981) *Developmental Programming for Infants and Young Children* (rev. ed.), University of Michigan, Ann Arbor, Michigan.

Sheehan, R. (1982) 'Infant Assessment: A Review and Identification of Emergent Trends,' in D. Bricker (ed.), *Intervention with At-Risk and Handicapped Infants: From Research to Application*, University Park Press, Baltimore.

Simeonsson, R.J., Huntington, G.S. and Parse, S.A. (1980) 'Assessment of Children with Severe Handicaps: Multiple Problems – Multivariate Goals,' *Journal of the Association for the Severely Handicapped*, 5(1), 55–72.

Slentz, K. (1986) *Evaluating the Instructional Needs of Young Children with Handicaps: Psychometric Adequacy of the Evaluation and Programming System: Assessment Level II (EPS-II)*, Unpublished doctoral dissertation, University of Oregon, Eugene.

Sparrow, S. S., Balla, D. A., and Cichetti, D. V. (1984) *Vineland Adaptive Behavior Scales*, American Guidance Service, Circle Pines, Minnesota.

Stevens, J. and King, E. (1976) *Administering Early Childhood Programs*, Little, Brown and Co., Boston.

Uzgiris, I. and Hunt, J.McV. (1975) *Assessment in Infancy: Ordinal Scales of Psychological Development*, University of Illinois Press, Urbana.

Vietze, P. M. and Coates, D. (1986) 'Using Information Processing Strategies for Early Identification of Mental Retardation,' *Topics in Early Childhood Special Education*, 6(3), 72–85.

FOOTNOTE

1. Support for this chapter was provided by Grants Number G008400661 and G008630372 from the US Office of Education to the Centre on Human Development.

8 PARENT INVOLVEMENT

Garry Hornby

INTRODUCTION

Parents have a key role in early intervention for their infants with
special needs. There are several reasons for this. First, without
active involvement of parents the developmental progress made
by children will typically be reduced. Second, unless the intervention has some impact on parents themselves it is unlikely that gains
which the children make will be maintained in the long term
(Guralnick and Bennett, 1987). Finally, since the improvement of
family functioning as a whole is a goal of early intervention, the
needs of parents for support and guidance must be a major
consideration (Fewell and Vadasy, 1986).

This chapter will discuss various aspects of parent involvement of relevance to professionals concerned with early intervention. These include: the process of adaptation to the disability; the
early needs of parents; models of family functioning; a model of
parent involvement; one example of parent-professional partnership; and the skills, attitudes and knowledge needed by professionals in order to work effectively with parents.

ADAPTATION PROCESS

A myriad of different models have been proposed to explain the
process which parents experience in adapting to their child's
disability (for example, Seligman, 1979; Wright, Granger and Sameroff, 1984). Most writers describe a stage model of adaptation
to loss, similar to the one proposed by Hornby (1982), which is
outlined below. Feedback on this model, from a large number of

parents and professionals, has confirmed its value in elucidating the process. Although there is some debate among professionals as to the accuracy of such a stage model, it has been this writer's experience that many parents gain considerable comfort from seeing such a conceptualization of the adaptation process.

The process of adaptation can be viewed as a continuum of reactions through which parents pass in order to come to terms with the disabling condition. The various reactions will now be described in the order in which they are typically experienced.

1. *Shock* — parents report feeling confusion, numbness, disorganization and helplessness. They often say that they were unable to take in much of what they were told at this time. This typically lasts from a few hours to a few days.

2. *Denial* — disbelief or denial of the reality of the situation often follows the shock reaction. As a temporary coping strategy this is quite healthy. However, prolonged denial can lead to parents shopping around for a more favourable diagnosis which, if pursued, could retard the adaptation process.

3. *Anger* — parents may search for a cause of the disability. They may blame themselves or hospital staff and experience anger which may be displaced onto their spouse, the child, or onto professionals involved. Underlying the anger may be feelings of guilt about producing an imperfect child.

4. *Sadness* — parents may feel depressed, despairing, or just very sad. This is often a reaction which pervades the whole process to some extent.

5. *Detachment* — many parents experience a time when they feel empty or flat. Nothing seems to matter. They accept the reality of the disability but have lost some of the meaning of life

6. *Reorganization* — this phase is characterized by realism and hope. Parents consider their 'cup is half-full rather than half-empty'.

7. *Adaptation* — when parents have come to terms with the situation they exhibit a mature emotional acceptance of the child with the disability.

In the adaptation phase they are fully aware of the child's special needs and strive to provide for these. However, the child is treated, as much as possible, as just another member of the family, which does not revolve around him or her. The parents may always experience some sadness that their child has a disability but they do not let this interfere with their efforts to make the best out of life.

The adaptation process is regarded as a normal, healthy reaction to the diagnosis of disability. Parents may need only a few days or take many years in which to work through this process. It can be viewed as a form of grieving similar to that which follows any traumatic loss.

Many parents have said that they experienced feelings associated with more than one phase at certain times. Some parents do not experience a particular phase, while others report being fixated at one phase for a considerable time before being able to move on. Some parents say that they experienced the phases in a different order. Thus, the process is qualitatively different for each parent and should be viewed only as a general guide and not as a prescription which all parents are expected to follow.Even after working through the continuum of reactions and having come to terms with the disability, parents are likely to experience sadness or grief which may always be present to some extent. This has led some writers to postulate that, rather than a grieving process which can be worked through with feelings to some extent resolved, parents of handicapped children experience 'chronic sorrow' (Olshansky, 1962; Wikler, Wasow, and Hatfield, 1981). It is suggested that the various reactions which are evoked, such as anger, sadness and denial, are not resolved but become an integral part of the parents' emotional life (Max, 1985). Thus, there will be numerous occasions when these reactions may be re-experienced. This reworking of parental reactions can occur at various milestones in the handicapped child's development such as school entry, the onset of puberty and leaving school. It can also occur when an additional disability is diagnosed at some time later than the original diagnosis.

An alternative way in which parental adaptation can be viewed has been proposed by Mitchell (1985). Parents are seen as progressing through a series of developmental stages, each of which is characterized by a set of tasks which must be at least partially mastered if parents are to adapt successfully to the presence of a handicapped person in the family. The four broad stages of development proposed are:

- initial diagnosis
- infancy and toddlerhood
- childhood and early adolescence
- late adolescence and adulthood

The tasks included in the first two stages, which are of greatest relevance to early intervention, are listed below.

Tasks associated with initial diagnosis

- deciding whether to pursue aggressive medical care where the infant's life is at risk
- deciding whether to keep the child or to seek institutionalization or adoption
- accepting the reality of the handicapping condition
- coming to terms with one's reactions to disability
- understanding the nature of the disability, its causation and developmental possibilities
- maintaining or enhancing self-esteem
- establishing a positive parenting relationship with the infant
- coming to terms with the reactions of family, friends and workmates
- maintaining or enhancing relationship with spouse

Tasks associated with infancy and toddlerhood

- making contact with other families with children with similar disabilities
- becoming familiar with and using appropriate support services
- establishing productive working relationships with particular professionals
- coping with reactions of the broader community

- becoming familiar with the rights of people with disabilities and their families, and acquiring advocacy skills
- establishing a balanced family and personal life
- developing competence in facilitating the child's development
- coping with the day-to-day tasks of caring for a child with a disability

The issue here is not whether parental adaptation should be viewed as a continuum of emotional reactions, or characterized by chronic sorrow, or by stages of developmental tasks. Each model is useful in providing professionals with some insight into the lives of these parents, thereby helping them to develop the understanding necessary for working with the families of children with special needs.

EARLY NEEDS OF PARENTS

Four important early needs of parents of children with disabilities are discussed below. These are: having the diagnosis of disability communicated to them in a sensitive and constructive manner; obtaining information about the handicapping condition and suggestions on facilitating the child's development; receiving emotional support and help in understanding feelings and reactions; and meeting other parents of children with similar disabilities.

Receiving the diagnosis

The vast majority of parents want to be told of the diagnosis by a professional who communicates empathy, sensitivity, openness, and a positive yet realistic outlook. This person should be knowledgeable about the possible causes and likely consequences of the disability and of the services available. Parents want to be told as soon as possible after the diagnosis is made, with both of them together and with the child present. They want to be told in a private place with no disturbances, and to have adequate time for information to be given, questions asked, and further interviews scheduled (Cunningham and Davis, 1985).

When the diagnosis is given in this way, parents tend to adapt more quickly and establish a more positive relationship with each other, the child and professionals (Cunningham and Glenn, 1985). However, many parents are still not given the diagnosis in this way (Hornby, 1987). These parents are almost always angry and resentful about the way they were told. This first, negative contact with a professional concerned with their handicapped child can sour their attitudes to future relationships with professionals. It therefore behoves all professionals to follow the above guidelines when communicating such information to parents.

Obtaining information

One of the very first requests of parents, after receiving the diagnosis, is for comprehensive, accurate and up-to-date information about their child's handicapping condition. Most parents also want suggestions as to how they can facilitate the child's development. Parents should also be told, at this time, about all the services and benefits available to help them care for their child with special needs. This information should be widely available in the form of both written materials and professional expertise. It is therefore quite alarming to discover how often it does not get to the parents.

Receiving support

Soon after the diagnosis parents need to have supportive counselling available to them. They need someone to help them express and clarify their feelings and to help in understanding their reactions and those of others around them. In this way parents can be assisted to make a speedy and successful adaptation to the situation. If they do not receive such counselling parents may experience considerable anguish and take much longer to move through the adaptation process. However, parents will seldom directly ask for counselling whereas they will ask for information on their child. Therefore, it is important for the person who supplies parents with this information to also have the skills necessary to carry out supportive counselling.

Meeting other parents

Surveys have shown that most parents want to meet others with similarly disabled children (Furneaux, 1988; Hornby, 1987). Whereas many parents wish to do this shortly after the diagnosis, some do not want such meetings for several months or even years. When parents do meet they typically report great benefits both in terms of obtaining information and in receiving support. One way of organizing such meetings is through the establishment of the parent-to-parent schemes which are described later in this chapter. Professionals can help to facilitate these contacts by making parents aware of the various support groups and other organizations, such as parent-to-parent schemes, operating in their area.

MODELS OF FAMILY FUNCTIONING

Several different models have emerged in recent years in the social sciences which have begun to have an impact on research and practice with families of children with special needs. Three of these are described below. These are: the transactional model; the ecological model; and family systems theory.

Transactional model

In this model development is believed to result from a continual interplay between a changing organism and a changing environment (Sameroff and Chandler, 1975). Thus, families are considered to both affect and be affected by their handicapped children. Also as children pass through different developmental stages they will affect their parents in different ways. For example, an infant with a disability will have a different effect on parents from an adolescent. Likewise, the effect parents have on their child with special needs will depend on the particular stage in the life cycle which they find themselves in. That is, a child with a handicapping condition who is the first born child of young, recently married parents is in a very different situation to a child with the same condition born to older parents who already have several other children.

Ecological model

In this model human development and behaviour cannot be understood independently of the context in which it occurs. Environment influences behaviour and this occurs at several levels (Bronfenbrenner, 1979). Thus, the effects on parents of caring for a child with special needs are strongly influenced by the environment in which they are living including the extended family, the services available and community attitudes. The family of a handicapped child is considered to constitute a microsystem with the child, parents and siblings reciprocally influencing each other. This family microsystem is influenced by the mesosystem in which it is embedded. The mesosystem comprises the range of settings in which the family actively participates, such as the extended family, school and work settings. The mesosystem is itself influenced by the exosystem. The exosystem level consists of settings in which the family is not actively involved but in which events occur that affect the family, such as the mass media, education system and voluntary agencies. Finally, there is the macrosystem which comprises the ideological systems inherent in the social institutions of a particular society such as religious, economic and political beliefs (Mitchell, 1985). Thus, the development and behaviour of a family with a handicapped child is influenced not only by interactions within its own microsystem but also by its interactions with other levels of the entire social system.

Family systems theory

In this model, the behaviour of family members is considered to be a function of the system of which they are a part. A change in the family system will inevitably lead to a change in the behaviour of each of the family members. Likewise, a change in an individual's behaviour will cause the family system to change. However, the functioning of the family system is considered to comprise more than just a summation of the contributions of its individual members. Intervention at the level of the family system is therefore likely to have more impact than intervention aimed at one of its members (Berger, 1984; Minuchin, 1974). The implication of this for professionals concerned with early intervention is that the whole family system needs to be considered when instituting a treatment programme — a point that has received considerable emphasis in American's PL 99-657.

In order to elucidate the various elements of the family system, a *Family Systems Conceptual Framework* has been developed by Turnbull and her associates (Turnbull, Summers, and Brotherson, 1984; Turnbull and Turnbull, 1986). This framework is made up of four components. First, there is the family interaction component which refers to the relationships that occur among and between the various sub-systems of family members. That is, the spousal sub-system (husband-wife interactions), the parent sub-system (parent-child interactions), and the sibling sub-system (child-child interactions). It also refers to extra-familial interactions such as those between children and grandparents or those between a father and his workmates.

Then, there is the family resources component which consists of descriptive elements of the family, including characteristics of the disability such as type and severity; characteristics of the family such as size, cultural background and socio-economic status; and personal characteristics such as health and coping styles.

The family functions component refers to the different types of needs which the family provides for, such as economic, physical care, recuperation, socialization, affection, self-definition, educational and vocational needs.

Finally, the family life cycle component represents the sequence of developmental changes that affect families as they progress through various stages in the life cycle, such as unattached adulthood, marriage, birth of children, school entry, adolescent children, children leaving home, and retirement. Family life cycle changes affect family functions and resources which in turn affect family interaction patterns. That is, the four components of the family system are interdependent. Therefore, the family systems approach suggests that an understanding of all four components of the family system is needed when considering the impact of an intervention on the family. The family systems conceptual framework also provides for the thorough analysis of families with handicapped children which should take place before an intervention is begun.

A MODEL FOR PARENT INVOLVEMENT

A model for parent involvement with parents of children with disabilities has been adapted from the work of Kroth (1985) and Lombana (1983). The model takes into account both parents' needs (what they require from professionals) and parents' strengths (what they can contribute). Included in the model is the assumption that whereas some needs or strengths apply to all parents others will only apply to a proportion of parents. The model describes four major strengths and four major needs of parents.

Strengths

Information — All parents can contribute valuable information about their child with special needs and about the family. Information concerning the child's strengths and weaknesses, likes and dislikes, along with relevant medical details can be gathered by professionals at the initial meeting. To gain an understanding of family resources, interaction, functions and life cycle stage may take further meetings. Making full use of this information is essential if interventions are to be effective. Professionals therefore need to develop good interviewing skills and a thorough understanding of the dynamics of exceptional families (Seligman, 1979).

Support — Most parents are willing and able to contribute more than just information. Most parents can support the efforts of professionals, in facilitating the development of their child with special needs, by reinforcing treatment procedures and by participating in planning the child's programme. Professionals therefore need to develop the skills of collaborating with parents in a parent-professional partnership (Mittler and McConachie, 1983).

Resource — Some parents have the ability and time to act as voluntary aides assisting with the intervention programme, in the preparation of materials, or provision of resources from the community. Others may have special skills which they can contribute such as in fundraising or helping prepare newsletters. Still others may have the time, skills and knowledge needed to provide support to other parents. Professionals should ensure that they make good use of this valuable resource (Michaelis, 1980).

Leadership — A few parents are able to provide training experiences for professionals through writing about their own experiences or speaking to groups such as teachers or doctors (Featherstone, 1981). Others may contribute their skills through executive membership of professional or parent organizations.

Needs

Communication — All parents need to have good communication with each of the professionals who is dealing with their child with special needs. They need to feel able to contact the relevant professional with any question or concern they may have. Also, all parents need to have up-to-date information about the various services and facilities which can help them care for their handicapped child. This can be provided by leaflets and handbooks written especially for parents (McConkey, 1985). However, professionals need to continually check that parents have received this information and are fully aware of all the services available to them.

Conferencing — Most parents want to be kept informed about their children's progress and to be given suggestions as to what they can do to help. They typically regard professionals involved in early intervention as a major source of information and support, and therefore need to have good working relationships with them. Professionals can facilitate this by maintaining regular contact with parents by telephone, mail or home visits. In addition, parents should be actively involved in any case conferences concerning their child with special needs. Professionals therefore need to be able to organize effective case conferences (Simpson, 1982).

Education — Many parents want to receive guidance from professionals in order to help them cope with their children's behaviour problems and facilitate their development (Harris, 1983; Topping, 1986). Such guidance, or parent training, can be organized individually, as in the Portage programme (White and Cameron, 1988), or in groups as with behavioural group training (Hornby and Singh, 1983). Group parent programmes can be designed to combine training with group counselling in order to provide a supportive environment in which parents can learn new skills and gain confidence through talking with other parents (Hornby and Murray, 1983). Likewise it has been acknowledged that professionals who provide such guidance individually should also combine it with the availability of counselling (White and Cameron, 1988). Therefore, in addition to the expertise of their own profession, early intervention personnel should also have good basic counselling skills.

Counselling — Some parents may need counselling beyond that which can be provided as part of the intervention programme. So, in addition to having basic counselling skills sufficient to deal with everyday concerns, early intervention personnel must be able to refer parents on to professional counsellors when the concerns raised would take them beyond their level of competence (Seligman, 1983; Webster, 1977). Some parents feel more at ease in individual counselling, others gain a great deal from participation in group counselling sessions (Hornby and Singh, 1982; Luterman, 1979). Therefore, it is important that professionals be aware of the various individuals and organizations in their community which can provide such counselling.

In this model of parent involvement adjectives such as 'most' and 'many' have been used to indicate different levels of strengths and needs. For example, whereas all parents can supply valuable information on their children, typically only a few are able and willing to play a leadership role. However, this is not to say that the opportunity to play a leadership role, or to act as a resource or support should not be extended to all parents. It is just that it should be accepted that, realistically, fewer parents can be expected to take up these roles. Likewise, although all parents need good communication with professionals and only some need professional counselling, it is still important to ensure that such counselling is made available to all parents.

The same can be said for parent training. Although the opportunity to receive training should be open to all parents, only a proportion of these will avail themselves of this. Both professionals and parents have cautioned against the overburdening of parents with a level of involvement in their children's developmental programmes which they cannot realistically maintain (Featherstone, 1981; Max, 1985). Parents ought to be able to opt for a level of involvement in the child's programme which is suitable to them at that time. Having offered a range of levels of involvement, professionals must accept that some parents, at some times, will choose to leave everything to the professionals while at other times they will want to be heavily involved (Baker, 1984). Both extremes should be possible within a flexible parent-professional partnership.

PARENT–PROFESSIONAL PARTNERSHIP

A partnership in which both parents and professionals share knowledge and skills in order to facilitate the child's development, and meet the needs of other family members is the best basis for parent involvement (Mittler and McConachie, 1983). One example of such a parent-professional partnership is described below in order to illustrate how parents and professionals can work together in setting up a service for parents of children with special needs. The following description of parent-to-parent schemes is also included in acknowledgement of the importance of such support groups in meeting some of the needs of parents for supportive counselling and up-to-date information.

Parent-to-parent schemes are support services for parents of children with special needs. Support is provided by a team of volunteer parents who themselves have children with similar needs. Enlightened professionals have long been aware of the value of putting parents in touch with one another. A parent-to-parent scheme simply develops this form of contact in a more organized way, and provides a form of support which is complementary to that offered by professionals.

Typically, parent-to-parent services operate as a telephone contact helpline. Schemes are advertised by means of leaflets, or posters put on notice-boards in places where parents are likely to see them, such as libraries, hospitals and schools. Parents seeking contact ring the helpline telephone number and are put in touch with a support parent who has a child with a similar disability. Parent-to-parent services were first established in the USA and have subsequently spread to Canada, Australia, New Zealand and the UK (Hornby, 1988; McConkey, 1985).

A principal feature of parent-to-parent services is the training of support parents. If professionals provide this training, a parent-professional partnership can form the basis of services. Thus, while professionals share their expertise in providing the training, it is the parents who provide support to other parents.

The parent-to-parent schemes in which the writer and his colleagues have been involved emphasized training parents in basic counselling skills (Hornby, 1988; Hornby, Murray, and Jones, 1987). Training courses are typically led by professionals skilled in group leadership and experienced in working with handicapped children and their families. Courses consist of eight, two-hour sessions beginning with two sessions in which parents share their experiences regarding their child with special needs. There are then five sessions in which parents learn basic counselling skills such as active listening, self-disclosure, and non-directive problem solving. The course concludes with a session on the organization of the parent-to-parent scheme.

Another feature of the schemes in which the writer has been involved is that they include parents of children with a wide range of disabilities. Through sharing experiences in their training groups, parents can see the similarities and differences in providing for children with different disabilities. Also, links are established between parents of children who have quite different disabilities, thus helping to break down the barriers which often exist between services for the different groups of handicapped children.

PROFESSIONAL KNOWLEDGE, ATTITUDES AND SKILLS

It is evident that there is certain knowledge, attitudes and skills which personnel involved with early intervention need to have over and above the expertise associated with their own professions.

Knowledge—Professionals should have a good understanding of the parental adaptation process and of the early needs of parents. When parents react to events with anger, denial or sadness, professionals should be able to be non-defensive and to help parents to work through their feelings, and thereby progress to a mature emotional acceptance of the child and his or her disability. Professionals should also have a thorough knowledge of the dynamics of families of children with special needs. This will enable interventions to be planned so that the functioning of such families is enhanced along with progress in the development of the handicapped child.

Attitudes — The attitudes which professionals require in order to work effectively with parents are ones which are consistent with the development of a productive partnership. To bring this about, professionals must possess the basic underlying attitudes of genuineness, respect and empathy (Rogers, 1980). They must be genuine in their relationships with parents. That is, they must come across as real people with strengths and weaknesses. For example, they should always be prepared to say that they 'don't know' when this is the case. In other words, they should relate to parents as people first and professionals second. Hiding behind a professional facade of competence is not in anyone's interest. Professionals should also show respect for parents. Parents' opinions and requests should always be given the utmost consideration. In the final analysis parents' wishes must be respected even if they run counter to the views of professionals. Most importantly, professionals should try to develop empathy with parents. They should be able to see the child and family's situation from the point of view of the parents. If professionals can develop an empathic understanding of the parents' position, then it is likely that a productive parent-professional partnership will evolve.

Skills — In order to work effectively with parents, professionals need good interpersonal communication skills. The most important part of this is the possession of basic counselling skills. Several authors have elaborated on the use of such skills with parents of children with special needs (Seligman, 1979; Turnbull and Turnbull, 1986). Briefly, what is required is the ability to: listen; understand; and help decide what action to take. Professionals must first of all listen to what parents have to say, in order to help them clarify their thoughts and feelings. Parents should then be helped to gain a clear understanding of the problem situation which they face or concern which they have. Finally, professionals should help parents decide what, if anything, they want to do about their problem or concern. That is, what action they wish to take. Possessing the skills required to implement this sample three-step problem-solving model of counselling will contribute enormously to the ability of professionals in establishing a productive working relationship with parents.

CONCLUSION

The most important variable in parent involvement is the relationship which professionals establish with parents. A positive, facilitative relationship is needed to promote constructive parent involvement. It is therefore important for professionals to develop a thorough understanding of the process of parental adaptation and of the needs of parents for support and guidance. Professionals should also be familiar with various models of family functioning as applied to families of children with special needs. They should also be aware of the range of methods for meeting parents' needs and utilizing their strengths which are suggested by a comprehensive model of parent involvement. Most importantly, professionals should develop a high level of interpersonal communication skills including sound basic counselling skills. These skills will promote the establishment of productive parent–professional partnerships which will in turn facilitate the effectiveness of early intervention programmes.

Summary of Major Comments and Recommendations

1. Parents have a key role in early intervention.

2. The process of parental adaptation to disability can be viewed as a continuum of reactions in a healthy process of re-adjustment.

3. Parents may be experiencing 'chronic sorrow'.

4. Parents can be considered to progress through a series of developmental stages, each characterised by a set of tasks.

5. Parents need to be told the diagnosis together, with the child present, in a private place, as soon as possible, by a professional who is sensitive and understanding.

6. Parents need comprehensive up-to-date information about their child's disability.

7. Supportive counselling should be available to parents from the diagnosis onward.

8. Most parents benefit from meeting other parents of children with similar disabilities.

9. Parents influence and are influenced by the behaviour of their handicapped children.

10. The effects on the family of caring for a handicapped child are strongly influenced by the environment in which the family lives.

11. The family can be considered to be a system with four important aspects: interaction; resources; functions; and life-cycle.

12. Parent involvement policy and practice is best guided by reference to an overall model which takes into account what parents can contribute as well as what they need.

13. Parent–to–parent schemes, organised so that professionals provide training and parents provide supportive counselling, are an example of parent–professional partnership.

14. In order to work effectively with parents, professionals should develop: attitudes of respect, genuineness and empathy; knowledge of the parental adaptation process and family dynamics; and the skills of effective interpersonal communication.

REFERENCES

Baker, B. L. (1984) 'Intervention with Families with Young, Severely Handicapped Children,' in J. Blacher (ed.), *Severely Handicapped Young Children and Their Families*, Academic Press, Orlando.

Berger, N. (1984) 'Social Network Interventions for Families that have a Handicapped Child,' in J. C. Hansen (ed.), *Families with Handicapped Members*, Aspen, Rockville.

Bronfenbrenner, U. (1979) *The Ecology of Human Development*, Harvard University Press, Cambridge, MA.

Cunningham, C. C. and Davis, H. (1985) *Working with Parents*, Open University Press, Milton Keynes.

Cunningham, C. C. and Glenn, S. M. (1985) 'Parent Involvement and Early Intervention,' in D. Lane and B. Stratford (eds), *Current Approaches to Down's Syndrome*, Holt, Rinehart and Winston, Eastbourne.

Featherstone, H. (1981) *A Difference in the Family*, Penguin, Harmondsworth.

Fewell, R. R. and Vadasy, P. F. (eds) (1986) *Families of Handicapped Children*, Pro-Ed, Austin.

Furneaux, B. (1988) *Special Parents*, Open University Press, Milton Keynes.

Guralnick, M. J. and Bennett, F. C. (eds) (1987) *The Effectiveness of Early Intervention for At-risk and Handicapped Children*, Academic Press, Orlando.

Harris, S.L. (1983) *Families of the Developmentally Disabled*, Pergamon, New York.

Hornby, G. (1982) 'Meeting the Counselling and Guidance Needs of Parents with Intellectually Handicapped Children,' *Mental Handicap in New Zealand*, 6, 8–27.

Hornby, G. (1987) 'Families with Exceptional Children,' in D. R. Mitchell and N. N. Singh (eds), *Exceptional Children in New Zealand*, Dunmore Press, Palmerston North.

Hornby, G. (1988) 'Launching Parent to Parent Schemes,' *British Journal of Special Education, 15,* (2), 77–78.

Hornby, G. and Murray, R. (1983) 'Group Programmes for Parents of Children with Various Handicaps,' *Child: Care, Health and Development, 9,* 185–198.

Hornby, G., Murray, R., and Jones, R. (1987) 'Establishing a Parent to Parent Service,' *Child: Care, Health and Development, 13,* 277–288.

Hornby, G. and Singh, N.N. (1982) 'Reflective Group Counselling for Parents of Mentally Retarded Children,' *British Journal of Mental Subnormality, 28,* 71–76.

Hornby, G. and Singh, N. N. (1983) 'Group Training for Parents of Mentally Retarded Children,' *Child: Care, Health and Development, 9,* 199–213.

Kroth, R. L. (1985) *Communicating with Parents of Exceptional Children (2nd ed.),* Love, Denver.

Lombana, J. H. (1983) *Home-school Partnerships,* Grune Stratton, New York.

Luterman, D. (1979) *Counselling Parents of Hearing Impaired Children,* Little Brown, New York.

Max, L. (1985) 'Parents' Views of Provisions, Services and Research,' in N. N. Singh and K. N. Wilton (eds), *Mental Retardation in New Zealand,* Whitcoulls, Christchurch.

McConkey, R. (1985) *Working with Parents,* Croom Helm, London.

Michaelis, C. T. (1980) *Home and School Partnership in Exceptional Education,* Aspen, Rockville.

Minuchin, S. (1974) *Families and Family Therapy,* Harvard University Press, Cambridge.

Mitchell, D. R. (1985) 'Guidance Needs and Counselling of Parents of Persons with Intellectual Handicaps,' in N. N. Singh and K. M. Wilton (eds), *Mental Retardation in New Zealand,* Whitcoulls, Christchurch.

Mittler, P. and McConachie, H. (eds) (1983) *Parents, Professionals and Mentally Handicapped People,* Croom Helm, London.

Olshansky, S. (1962) 'Chronic Sorrow: A Response to Having a Mentally Defective Child,' *Social Casework, 43,* 190–193.

Rogers, C. R. (1980) *A Way of Being,* Houghton Mifflin, Boston.

Sameroff, A. J. and Chandler, M. J. (1975) 'Reproductive Risk and the Continuum of Caretaking Casualty,' in F. D. Horowitz (ed.), *Review of Child Development Research, (Vol. 4),* University of Chicago Press, Chicago.

Seligman, M. (1979) *Strategies for Helping Parents of Exceptional Children*, Free Press, New York.

Seligman, M. (ed) (1983) *The Family with a Handicapped Child*, Grune and Stratton, New York.

Simpson, R. L. (1982) *Conferencing Parents with Exceptional Children*, Aspen, Rockville.

Topping, K. J. (1986) *Parents as Educators*, Croom Helm, London.

Turnbull, A. P., Summers, J. A. and Brotherson, M. J. (1984) *Working with Families with Disabled Members*, University of Kansas, Kansas.

Turnbull, A. P. and Turnbull, H. R. (1986) *Families, Professionals and Exceptionality*, Merrill, Columbus.

Webster, E. J. (1977) *Counselling with Parents of Handicapped Children*, Grune & Stratton, New York.

White, M. and Cameron, R. J. (eds) (1988) *Portage: Progress, Problems and Possibilities*, NFER-Nelson, Windsor.

Wikler, L., Wasow, M., and Hatfield, E. (1981) 'Chronic Sorrow Revisited,' *American Journal of Orthopsychiatry*, 51, 63–70.

Wright, J. S., Granger, R. D. and Sameroff, A. J. (1984) 'Parental Acceptance and Developmental Handicap,' in J. Blacher (ed.), *Severely Handicapped Young Children and Their Families*, Academic Press, Orlando.

9 MOTHER–CHILD INTERACTION AND EARLY LANGUAGE INTERVENTION

Penny Price and Sandra Bochner

INTRODUCTION

The importance of the close relationship between mother and child in infancy has been recognized for centuries, but only more recently have studies of the effects of disruption to this basic bond been investigated in detail. In a comprehensive review of research in this area, Mitchell (1987) describes the effects of disruption on premature infants, deaf infants, abused infants and developmentally delayed infants. Disruption can take the form of physical separation, as in the case of children born very prematurely, or it can be disruption to the normally developing interaction patterns which results from very passive or very disruptive behaviour on the part of the child, which leaves the parent without feedback to his or her interactive attempts, and may in time cause the parent to cease interacting with the child other than in the most limited manner. This lack of synchrony between mother and child in earliest infancy can have long-lasting effects on the child's developing communication skills — a subject which has given rise to an extensive research effort in recent years, and to which further reference will be made later in the chapter.

The purpose of the first part of this chapter is to review the theoretical influences which have shaped current practice, and to examine some of the issues related to the involvement of parents in early intervention, with a particular focus on the role of the mother or primary caregiver in facilitating and mediating early learning in disabled and high-risk infants through ongoing interaction with their infants. In the second part of the chapter, some recent theoretical and research findings are described in relation to their effect on the development of early language intervention programming. Some language programmes are described in detail and some guidelines for future practice are outlined. The third section of the chapter presents a set of conclusions.

CONTEMPORARY PERSPECTIVE ON CHILD DEVELOP-MENT AND MOTHER–CHILD INTERACTION

Current explanations about the processes that underlie development in early childhood vary in the relative emphasis given to the role of the mother or primary caregiver in the developmental process. These variations can be recognized in many of the teaching programmes currently used in early intervention services. In reviewing some of the more influential of the explanations or 'theories' about child development and mother–infant interaction, two questions can be asked.

1. What processes are involved in early development?

2. What is the contribution of mother–infant interaction to the developmental process?

In the following section of this chapter, four theoretical explanations of infant development will be examined in terms of these questions. The answers that are found should provide a basis upon which decisions can be made about the possible contributions of social interaction, particularly mother–infant interaction, to the educational process inherent in early intervention programmes. The focus of this discussion will be limited in two ways: first, the examination of explanations of development will be primarily concerned with the areas of cognition and language, since these areas appear to be more crucially affected by mother–child interaction than other areas of development. Secondly, reference will be made, primarily, to explanations based on studies of children who are developing normally, since most of the research in this area has been concerned with these groups. However, consideration will also be given to the relevance of these theories for infants and children who have developmental delays or disabilities.

The four theoretical explanations of development to be considered here have been termed: Nativist, Behavioural, Cognitive, Interactive. Each will be discussed in terms of the contribution of a few representative theorists.

NATIVIST THEORY (e.g. Bower, 1971; Chomsky, 1965)

What processes underlie early development?

Explanations of the Nativist type assert that there is a biological basis to infant development. For example, Bower and others argue that neonatal responses to human stimuli are inborn and function as a mechanism for survival. Their studies of speech detection (Eimas and Tartter, 1979) demonstrate, they claim, that from birth, infants show evidence of an innate awareness of 'humanness'. They suggest that there are innate 'social stimulus feature detectors' which enable very young infants to respond to multidimensional social stimuli like faces and voices before they are able to respond to information from single modalities such as photographs of a face or a single speech contrast.

Such examples demonstrate that at the earliest stage of development infants are innately responsive to humans, having, in the area of social development, relatively high levels of 'abstract' skills that, over time, become increasingly specific. This developmental trend, from highly abstract or general to increasingly specific social knowledge, is exemplified in the fear of strangers response commonly exhibited by infants during their first year (Bronson, 1978; Brooks and Lewis, 1976; Fagan, 1976). Over time, most babies develop highly individualized communication patterns with familiar adults, particularly the primary caregiver, so that by seven months or so, they are able to distinguish a stranger and become fearful, particularly if the stranger attempts to interact with them.

A similar viewpoint is taken by theorists such as Chomsky (1965), a psycholinguist noted for his work on children's acquisition of language. Along with others (e.g. Lenneberg, 1967; McNeill, 1970), Chomsky argues for the existence of a Language Acquisition Device (LAD), a structure inherent within the child which provides a broad framework for language. The specific form of the language is gained through contact with the adult language system used in the child's immediate environment. The fact that most children master the essentials of their language — an enormously complex task — before they enter school at the age of four or five years, and that the developmental pattern of early language acquisition has universal features, is used by Chomsky and other Nativists to justify their theory of an innate mechanism for language acquisition.

What is the contribution of mother–child interaction to the developmental process?

According to Nativist theorists, developmental change results primarily from maturational factors within the child rather than from the influence of environmental factors such as social interaction. Bower and his associate (1979) argue that infants are born with an innate and unusually advanced responsiveness to humans, and that the task of the primary caregiver is to ensure that development occurred as expected. In a discussion of this issue, at a pediatric conference, Bower and Wishart stated:

> I think babies come into the world better prepared than
> we are willing to give them credit for ... They respond
> immediately to adult speech with social behaviour.
> Obviously the world must be a very confusing place for
> them, but they already have some sort of built-in
> structure that programs them to organize it in a human
> way. A sort of biological safeguard ... They are getting
> new input all the time. That new input has to be
> reorganized on the basis of what's gone before.
> Development is not just additive. It's a matter of
> direction to start with. Any amount of later intervention
> is futile if you don't know which developmental path
> he's taken in the first place. (Bower and Wishart, 1979, p.
> 88f)

The role of the mother is to model correct sentences so that the child, the active agent in the developmental process, can develop hypotheses about the rules that govern language.

Explanations of infant development based on innate mechanisms are relatively pessimistic about the contribution that can be made by social agents to the developmental process. Their role is important in providing opportunities for the child to acquire developmentally appropriate behaviour, in the form of attending to human rather than non-human stimuli, and in acquiring culturally appropriate knowledge in the form of the specific language of their community. The role of the adult is, however, secondary to the biological mechanism within the infant in terms of the developmental process.

BEHAVIOURIST THEORY (e.g. Skinner, 1957; Mowrer, 1954)

What processes underlie early development?

In contrast to the relatively passive role attributed to caregivers by nativist theorists, behaviourists take a far more positive view of the contribution that is made by adults to the developmental process. This explanation has been termed 'empirical' because it was derived, initially, from laboratory studies of learning in animals, and later, from systematic observation of children's behaviour in the early stages of learning.

Explanations of early development classified as 'behavioural' vary from those based on simple stimulus–response associations (e.g. the baby gurgles and the mother reinforces this act by tickling, smiling and murmuring) to more complex mechanisms. For example, Braine (1963) used the process of stimulus–response generalization to explain the appearance of grammatically correct sentence forms in children's speech. Skinner (1957), one of the most frequently cited behavioural theorists, explained language development in terms of an operant model of learning. According to this view, infants learn to talk by being rewarded (reinforced) by mothers or caregivers for vocalizations that often appear to be produced spontaneously (i.e. without an apparent stimulus). Skinner identified three main types of operant vocal behaviour in infants: a mand (or command) as, for example, in the previously cited example when the infant gurgles, perhaps to attract attention, and the caregiving adult responds with a touch and a word; a tact (or comment) as when the infant gurgles at the sight of a mobile and the mother responds by activating the toy and commenting on what is happening; and an echoic utterance, which occurs when an infant imitates the sounds that have just been produced by a caregiver, who, in turn, responds by praising this attempt at speech.

A slightly different explanation of early language development from a behavioural viewpoint, but based on the same process, was proposed by Mowrer (1958) who suggested that infants initially learn to make speech sounds by imitating the sounds produced by mother at a time that was highly pleasurable for both (e.g. at bathtime or getting ready for bed). During a bath, mother might repeat the word 'quack' several times, as part of a game with a toy duck, and the infant echoes the word. Later, during playful babbling alone in the cot, the infant recognizes this sound in the string of vocalizations and repeats it, remembering with pleasure its association with the game in the bath. Mowrer argues that such self-reinforcing practice establishes neural and muscular patterns that provide a basis for language acquisition.

In contrast to the nativist viewpoint described earlier, the behaviourists see the contribution of environmental influences, and the role of mother–child interaction, as an important factor in child learning.

What is the contribution of mother–infant interaction to the developmental process?

Behaviourists argue that new skills can be learned by a process of 'chaining' or linking new behaviours to those that have already been acquired. So the trigger, or 'cue', for a new vocal behaviour can be embedded in an old one, as, for example, when the child learns, through appropriate reinforcement, to associate 'duck' with the previously learned utterance 'quack' and then learns, again as a result of appropriate reinforcement, to add 'gone' to 'duck' to signal the game in which the toy duck disappears under the bath water.

Critics of behavioural explanations of early development point out that the rate of acquisition of skills in children who are developing normally is too rapid to be adequately explained in terms of stimulus–response associations. Moreover, the behavioural model does not explain novel or untrained behaviours. Nor does it adequately explain non-observable aspects of behaviour, such as language comprehension and cognitive skills. However, behavioural models of learning do attribute a critical role to the mother or caregiver, as the reinforcing agent, and this has important implications for early intervention. Whereas the nativist view attributes little value to the role of the mother in early development, behavioural explanations place responsibility for generating behaviour change squarely upon the mother or consistent caregiver, both in relation to the pairing of responses and rewards to reinforce desirable behaviour, and in relation to modelling and shaping behaviours by appropriate stimulus reinforcement.

A number of the early intervention programmes (Hayden and Dimitriev, 1975; Heber and Garber, 1975; Shearer and Shearer, 1976) adopted a behavioural approach and many of these programmes proved to be highly effective in teaching specific skills to children with disabilities. However, problems were encountered in the generalization of these skills to situations outside the often highly restricted classroom situation. These difficulties were particularly evident in the area of language skills: children could be taught to produce quite complex grammatical utterances in a one-to-one setting, but there was often no evidence that they used these newly acquired skills to communicate spontaneously with their family or peers. Moreover, both educators and parents were often uneasy about the use of highly structured, tightly controlled, behavioural teaching techniques that were, in many respects, incompatible with the modes of interactions that occurred naturally in home and classroom. Gradually, interest turned to other explanations of early development, particularly to those proposed by Piaget and others who focused on the contribution of cognitive development to the acquisition of language and other related skills, and to the place of social interaction in facilitating development among children with disabilities.

COGNITIVE THEORY (e.g. Piaget, 1978; Werner and Kaplan, 1964)

What processes underlie early development?

Piaget was primarily interested in the development of children's thinking. He saw it in terms of four main stages, involving a progression from the earliest sensorimotor stage, when the infant learns about the world by direct action on objects, to the final stage of formal operations, when the person is capable of formal or abstract thought. Earliest knowledge is gained as infants look, grasp and suck objects and entities that come within their reach. Through these experiences, both knowledge about the properties of objects and strategies for exploring them are acquired. Over time, babies develop concepts about things they have encountered, such as an idea about the 'roundness' of balls, or a knowledge that 'mother' represents comfort, and security. According to Piaget, developmental change occurs when infant knowledge about an entity or event is challenged, when children encounter something (e.g. a 'square ball') that is inconsistent with their previous experience and knowledge. This situation is termed 'disequilibrium' by Piaget who then argued that the children's task in this situation is to modify or change the concept they hold so that it can 'accommodate' this new knowledge (e.g. that some balls are square, or that mother can, at times, be angry) into the relevant concept. It is by means of this process of taking in new information and integrating it into existing knowledge that cognitive development takes place. Language, according to Piaget, provides a symbolic system by which children can represent what they know at times when the actual objects or events are not there. So, according to this view of early development, children's knowledge of the world emerges from their experiences and language provides a means of representing what is known.

A slightly different approach to the study of cognitive and language development was taken by Werner and Kaplan (1964). Like Piaget, they also rejected the nativist and behavioural explanations that were dominant at that time. They attempted, in their work, to integrate two distinct ideas about language and thought, one 'holistic' or focusing on the whole situation in which children develop, and the other developmental, based on the assumption that the developmental process involves a progression from relatively simple to increasingly complex behaviour. They argued that, initially, infants are unable to distinguish between themselves and objects in the environment, but, over time, they learn to differentiate between themselves and objects that they can touch and see around them. However, unlike Piaget who was concerned with the cognitive processes ongoing within the child, Werner and Kaplan argued that the early awareness of objects in infancy, and the differentiation of object from self is dependent upon the child being within a close nurturing relationship with a caregiver. In such a situation, infants are free from anxiety and able to attend to those aspects of the environment that impinge upon them.

What is the contribution of mother–infant interaction to the developmental process

According to Piaget, acquisition and absorption of new information into previously acquired knowledge are processes that children have to experience for themselves. Others, including, of course, mothers, fathers, and siblings, cand help by involving the infants in experiences that exceed what they have previously encountered. Adults can play a facilitative role, by encouraging the children to attend to relevant aspects of an event (e.g. the square ball can be thrown or hit). However, the contribution that can be made by adults to infant cognitive development is, essentially, very limited.

While Piaget's model of early development has been highly influential in early intervention, uncertainty about some aspects of his theory, particularly in relation to his emphasis on objects rather than people, and on the relationship he proposed between early cognitive and language development, led to an interest in explanations that focused more precisely on the contribution of children's social experiences to their early development.

This change in emphasis is evident in the work of Werner and Kaplan (1964) who placed much greater emphasis on the social bases of language acquisition than Piaget, asserting that linguistic symbols emerge from the child's shared attention with an adult, to an entity that attract their interest. They saw three critical elements in the emergence of language: the child and his or her partner (i.e. communicator and communicatee), the topic of their shared interest (object, entity or activity) and the symbols (signs, words) used to designate this topic. The influence of this focus on the contribution of social aspects of children's cognitive and social development is developed more fully in the final theoretical explanation to be considered here — the interactional or transactional approach.

INTERACTIVE THEORY (e.g., Bruner, 1977; Sameroff, 1975; Vygotsky, 1962)

What processes underlie early development?

Whereas Piaget was primarily concerned with cognitive development, focusing on the processes within children that contributed to change, others, such as Bruner, Vygotsky, Sameroff and McLean and Snyder-MacLean (1978), also placed value on the contribution of caregivers to the development of early cognitive and language skills. For example, Bruner writes about the 'scaffolding' that adults provide for children's development, as they stimulate, reinforce, model and prompt children during face-to-face games and other activities. Bruner describes the interactive or reciprocal games that mothers and their infants play, repeating the actions innumerable times (particularly during the early months when the infant's responses are limited to primitive vocalizations), looking and reaching. He emphasizes the importance of adult modelling of actions that match the child's developmental level, and of the development of 'joint actions' and 'joint reference' between infant-adult pairs.

Vygotsky, writing in the 1920s and 1930s was mainly interested in language as a determinant of intellectual development, and the contribution of social experiences, specifically interaction between adults and children, to the process of developmental change. Vygotsky conceptualized the 'zone of proximal development' as a way of describing the difference between what a child can do without help, and what can be achieved under the guidance of an adult or more capable peer. According to this view, developmental change occurs as a result of 'tutoring' by a more experienced or knowledgeable person. This is a more extreme version of explanations of early development that place some emphasis on the role of influences within the social environment. For example, Sameroff (1975) argued that significant members of a child's family (i.e., those who interact frequently with the child) can have as much influence upon the developmental process as factors internal to the child. The idea of a mutually interactive process underlying development is also evident in McLean and Snyder-McLean's (1978) 'transactional' model of language development. They suggest that infants must enter into a 'language-learning partner-ship with mature language users'. This view of development provides a very positive framework within which early interven-tion programmes can be devised.

What is the contribution of mother–infant interaction to the developmental process?

Clearly, the interactive explanations of development attribute an important role to mother or caregiver–child interaction in the developmental process. However, the relative weight given to the contribution of each member of the dyad can vary. For example, Bruner gives equal value to each, particularly as the infant moves out of the neonatal stage. He describes such interaction in terms of reciprocal exchanges, emphasizing the need for the infant to become an active participant in this relationship. Any disturbance in the development of such a relationship between mother–infant pairs, as in the case of severe impairment in the infant or an extreme disturbance in the mother, could pose a threat to the developmental process and compensatory measures may need to be introduced to overcome any such threats to the developing child. Vygotsky, on the other hand, focuses on the contribution that can be made by the mother, or tutor, to the developmental process. According to this viewpoint, the mother/tutor has the potential to maximize the pace of development by providing appropriate activities for the child and guiding him or her towards higher levels of performance. However, there are also limits on the extent to which a tutor can increase a child's rate of learning. As the discrepancy between actual and potential developmental lev-els diminishes, progress inevitably decreases. Further, the concept of the 'zone of proximal development' does not identify proce-dures whereby changes in children's potential developmental levels can be promoted.

SUMMARY

Each of the models discussed has something to contribute to our understanding of the factors that underlie early development in children, and the place of mother-child interaction in this process. The models vary in the relative importance ascribed to the contribution of mother and child in the developmental process, and in the processes identified as being significant for the acquisition of new skills.

In the following section the changing theoretical view–points, combined with research evidence on various aspects of language acquisition, including the importance of mother–child interaction, will be related to developments in early language intervention programming.

EARLY LANGUAGE INTERVENTION PROGRAMMES

The search for effective language intervention procedures has become one of the major tasks for those involved with the provision of education and other services for young children with developmental delays and other handicapping conditions. Unprecedented growth has taken place in this area of endeavor in the last two decades, and is likely to continue into the 1990s. The problems faced by those involved in the provision of services have been confounded by the constantly shifting focus of research into the nature and process of early language acquisition, and by the fact that results of research studies have often provided conflicting information and conclusions. Although the clear guidelines sought by interventionists for incorporation into language programmes have been elusive, progress has been and continues to be impressive. These issues will be reviewed in some detail in the next sections of this chapter.

Theory and Research Evidence — Influences on Developing Early Language Intervention Programmes

Anastasiou (1981), in his review of two decades of early intervention programming, comments that the theoretical bases of programmes have changed over time, in line with the changing

237

explanations for early development which were reviewed above. The nativist viewpoint has never given rise to early intervention programmes. If it is believed that a child does not have the innate capacity to learn, then no amount of environmental manipulation will alter the situation. The fervour with which behavioural theories were translated into intervention programmes perhaps reflected the relief experienced by those concerned with the development and welfare of developmentally delayed and slow learning children at finding an optimistic approach which stated that learning is directly affected by the manipulation of environmental factors. Programmes using behavioural principles were established, covering all areas of development — motor, cognitive, language, social and emotional skills, and aimed at children from infancy through to school age, with home-based programmes, centre-based programmes and a combination of the two. Satisfactory results were achieved in teaching the acquisition of many skills. Programmes tended to be adult-dominated, with the child viewed as a passive learner, responding to carefully chosen stimuli, and reinforced with a variety of extrinsic reinforcers in some cases combined with social praise. Over a period of time, it was observed that problems with this approach emerged in the area of generalization, with skills that had been taught in clinical settings failing to generalize into natural usage in the child's everyday life. A further problem was the denial of the child's active role in the learning process. Cognitive psychologists, working with young children in a variety of capacities, observed that they appeared to learn best through active participation and that interaction with objects and people in their environment, and that only those things which were meaningful to the child were learned and maintained and transferred into regular usage.

Reviews of behavioural research in the mid 1970s (Garcia and de Haven, 1974; Snyder and Mclean, 1976) encouraged recognition of the fact that certain skills were appropriately taught by this technology (especially motor skills and some self-help skills), whereas others such as language, social and cognitive skills required a more interactive framework for successful acquisition. Extensive research into factors and processes affecting early language acquisition supported the finding that behavioural procedures were not the most suitable for facilitating this most crucial of all skills at the preschool level. Early research into language acquisition focused on the syntactic system, and behavioural programmes used this knowledge for the content of their programmes which were taught by means of behavioural procedures.

Research into the semantic, pragmatic and discourse aspects of communication led to major changes in the content of language programmes, the settings in which they were implemented, the personnel involved in implementation and the procedures and activities involved. Language could no longer be viewed as an abstract system, unrelated to the child's particular environment (Chomsky, 1957). The child's earliest communications preceded the capacity to use words, and taxonomies of pragmatic intent were developed (Halliday, 1976; McConkey and Price, 1986) which could be used to facilitate understanding of the earliest communicative attempts made by infants. Semantic categories, developed by psycholinguistic researchers such as Bloom (1973), Bowerman (1973) and Nelson (1973) provided a way of analyzing children's earliest utterance in terms of the child's conceptual holdings about his or her environment and the relationships within it. It was found that the order in which these concepts were encoded in language was uniform across cultures, suggesting that language is dependent upon cognition for its earliest form and content.

Research into the 'discourse' features of communication has emphasized the social and interactive aspects of language and has led to a changed interpretation of the purpose of the features which characterize interaction between caregivers and their young children. The 'fine-tuning' theory which states that mothers modify their speech for the specific purpose of 'teaching' their children language (Moerk, 1976) and that they achieve this by progressively modelling the language that the child needs to hear in order to acquire the increasingly complex syntactic structures of their native language, has not been supported by research evidence and is no longer widely held (Price, 1988). Rather, the research evidence of Snow, Perlmann and Nathan (1985), Wells (1980, 1981, 1985) and others has lent support to the responsiveness theory which states that the purpose of mother speech is to involve the child in conversation. Only in conversation does the child learn all the facets of the linguistic system. By providing a conversational framework which allows for immature skills, the child is involved in meaningful interaction through which he or she gradually learns the discourse, pragmatic, semantic and syntactic skills of the mature language user. The child can attend to and incorporate those features which are appropriate to his or her stage of conceptual, social and linguistic growth, while the mother sustains the conversation. So the changes in maternal speech result from the development of the child's ability to take his or her turn in the conversation.

A review of research into the semantic, pragmatic and social bases of language led Mclean and Snyder-McLean (1978) to formulate a transactional model of early language acquisition which emphasizes the importance of interacting cognitive, linguistic and social factors, and states that unless children have a reason to communicate and someone meaningful to communicate with, they will not learn to talk. McLean and Snyder-McLean's review and evaluation of language intervention programmes in terms of how adequately they incorporated the essential cognitive, social and linguistic bases of knowledge have had a significant effect on the development of language intervention programmes in the last decade. So, too, have the major findings from mother–child interaction research. From these we have learned that adjustments in maternal speech, aimed at providing a simplified syntactic model for the child, are not facilitatory, unlike semantic, pragmatic and discourse adjustments which ensure the child's participation in conversational exchange (Bellinger, 1980; Cross, 1981). We have learned that it is essential to look at the behaviour of both partners in the interaction, an important finding for the development of intervention procedures where frequently the focus is either on the child or the mother (Conti-Ramsden, 1985). We have learned from Wells (1985) that engaging the child in conversation about the immediate situation, and the joint activity which occurs when mother and child are involved in routine everyday tasks in their natural setting, can result in rapid language development. This emphasis on the cognitive and social bases of language, on the active role of the child and on the crucial nature of the interaction between child and caregiver has resulted in a shift in intervention programming from clinical to natural settings. In addition parents rather than clinicians have become the intervenors with preschool teachers being involved in the facilitation partnership. There has also been a shift in focus from syntactic structures to an emphasis on child-generated semantic and pragmatic content based on the activities and purposes relevant to the child's cognitive level and social environment.

The changes that have occurred in language intervention procedures are evidence of the fact that theoretical formulation and empirical evidence do have a continuing and desirable impact on practice. The review of programmes which follows will illustrate this point further. Programmes vary in their theoretical foundations and in their capacity to respond to changing ideas about language acquisition, but sensitivity to new perspectives and the flexibility to incorporate them into programming procedures may be one of the most important factors differentiating the merely adequate from the excellent.

REVIEW OF SELECTED EARLY LANGUAGE INTERVENTION PROGRAMMES

This review of programmes is not comprehensive, but, attempts to illustrate some of the more important developments which have taken place in the last decade, and reflect the directions discussed in the previous section. Some programmes which were strongly behavioural in orientation have modified their procedures in the light of research findings in the area of semantics and pragmatics. Others were developed from within a transactional or interactional framework. Some have been implemented within pre-school or centre-based programmes and others have been employed exclusively with parents and their young children, either individually or in groups. Others have combined parent and classroom programmes. Programmes which have developed from a behavioural framework tend to have a more structured approach to goal setting, teaching procedures and data collection. There is a discernible trend towards a less structured approach with more emphasis on spontaneous interaction with an understanding of the responsive role that the adult plays in language acquisition. The work of Hart and Risley (1974) and Hart and Rogers-Warren (1978) exemplify the modifications made to a basically behaviourist approach, which was initially concerned with teaching syntactic structures. The necessity for teaching language relevant to the child in natural settings, in order to ensure generalization, led to the development of what they termed 'incidental' teaching in pre-school settings, targeting functional language and making access to toys, teaching attention and other classroom activities contingent upon individually determined child verbalizations. Developments in their work have continued into the 1980s.

Another programme is the TELL (Teach Early Language for Living) developed in the Down's Programme at Macquarie University (Cairns *et al.*, 1982. It has its roots in a behaviourist tradition but has been developed using McLean and Snyder-McLean's transactional model for its content and environmental setting. This programme has specific assessment procedures in the areas of pragmatics, imitation skills, semantics and syntactics, comprehension and articulation. It also sets specific goals and requires data to be kept on the specified number of trials for each item. But the goals targeted are selected on the basis of environmental relevance and are targeted in a variety of natural situations within the preschool day, as well as during specific language teaching sessions. Parents are involved, carrying targets into the home situation. The programme is detailed and prescriptive, but does emphasize the importance of natural targets in natural environments using natural, communication-related reinforcers.

The programme of Bricker and Carlson (1980) has been developed within the framework of a long-running early intervention programme. It pays particular attention to the prerequisite social and cognitive or sensorimotor skills of the prelinguistic period, and consists of a two-tiered lattice system which specifies in detail the social and cognitive skills essential for the development of referential behaviour and verbal language. Bricker and Carlson's decision to programme for intervention from earliest infancy was in response to the emphasis in the literature upon the crucial importance of the prelinguistic period for the development of communication.

A programme which was evaluated by McLean and Snyder-McLean (1978) as incorporating more features of their transactional model than any other currently available programme was the Environmental Language Intervention Programme (ELIP) developed by MacDonald *et al.* (1974). The ELIP is a comprehensive package containing assessment procedures covering the child's use of language in the home, the parents' attitude to the child's problem, the child's preverbal skills and verbal skills assessed in terms of semantic grammatical rules. A handbook suggests a format for weekly intervention sessions over a period of 12 weeks. The programme differs from its predecessors in its emphasis on ensuring the adequate development of preverbal skills before targeting verbal skills. One and two word utterances are assessed in terms of semantic-relational categories, which are developed in structured and then semi-structured play routines with parents taking the role normally adopted by clinicians. Parents are viewed as real partners in the intervention process, selecting suitable goals for language targets in terms of the child's needs in their home environment. Instructions to parents on desirable modifications of their language when interacting with their child are limited to ensuring that the child is attending, that language used is clear and simple and restricted to classes of words that the child is learning, and to encouraging expansions and comments — a mixture of suggestions stemming from mother–child interaction research to date. This work, developed at the Nisonger Centre in Ohio, USA, has been instrumental in stimulating intervention programs in both Canada and Australia. MacDonald's (1985) recent work has involved the development of a model for developing communication skills in severely delayed children. The model attempts to analyze the variables involved in the child, the significant adult with whom he or she is interacting, and the setting. The primary goal is to increase the length of participation in turn-taking interactions, reflecting the current concern with facilitating language growth through participation in conversational discourse in the child's natural environment. Results of this approach are not yet available but the model may well prove to be a valuable addition to the predominantly behavioural procedures currently used with severely and profoundly retarded persons.

The ELIP was developed at the Macquarie University Special Education Centre in Sydney, Australia, in response to a request to fill a gap in the early intervention services available to young developmentally delayed children (Bochner, Price and Salamon, 1982). An initial parent training project was established based on the assessment and training procedures developed by Horstmeier and MacDonald (1975). Since 1980, the programme has been operating in community health centres as well as the University Special Education Centre. It has assisted several hundred children and their parents, as well as providing training for students, pre-school teachers and other professionals involved with the education of young developmentally delayed children. The programme has undergone considerable modification, with particular emphasis being placed on the skills required at the prelinguistic stage. These include looking together, turn-taking, and appropriate play with objects and people for they are the building blocks for language development. The original section on how mothers talk to their children, emphasizing the necessity for responsiveness, extending the child's language and providing him or her with plenty of opportunity, has been extended to include the importance of turn-taking, and extending the number of turns in a conversational sequence. In addition to suggesting games and activities appropriate to the home setting for skills ranging from preverbal to early sentences, the programme includes suggestions for group activities which allow for the participation of children at differing levels of language skill. A series of video-tapes illustrates how to assess the child's level and demonstrates suitable strategies and activities for encouraging language growth.

Research reports have substantiated the overall effectiveness of the programme, with gains on the SICD (Sequenced Inventory of Communication Development, Hedrick, Prather and Tobin, 1965) demonstrating growth over six months at a rate comparable to that of normal language learning children (Price and Bochner, 1984; Bochner *et al.*, 1986). But global measures fail to provide information about which aspects of the programme are effective for which children at which stage of development. An early attempt to investigate changes in patterns of interaction between ten mothers and their developmentally delayed children over the six month period of the language programme provided strong evidence of an increase in child turn-taking and a reduction in the amount that mothers talked. Very tentative evidence suggested that a continued high usage of directives unaccompanied by commenting and feedback may be associated with slow language growth in children at the 2+ word level. The shortcomings of this study, which did not allow analysis within a discourse framework, led to the development of a longitudinal study which is attempting to look at changes in discourse patterns over an 18 month period. The study is particularly concerned with investigating how joint attention is negotiated between mother and child, what causes breakdown and how this is resolved. It is hoped that analysis of breakdown situations may lead to the development of suggestions and strategies which may be specifically, rather than generally, applicable to mothers who experience this problem, usually with children who are difficult to engage in joint activity and have very short attention spans. An analysis of correction strategies, ranging from direct to indirect, is being examined in relation to patterns of initiating and responding behaviour and it is hoped to shed further light on the conversational versus directive style controversy. The study will also yield information about changing patterns of discourse features as they relate to different contexts and to stages of language development in children with different levels of retardation.

A more recent development at Macquarie University is the establishment of a programme which combines parent training and home intervention with a classroom based component which focuses on the child's use of language in social situations with other children and adults, and explores the effect of different contexts within the classroom on communicative behaviour (Bochner, 1987). The children are assessed and then attend a pre-school classroom for two mornings a week in which every aspect of the programme is designed to facilitate the development of communication and social skills on either an individual or a small group basis. Parents attend group sessions one morning a week, discuss issues relevant to early language acquisition and the adult's role in acquisition. They observe their children in the classroom, discuss the language level their child is at and plan the most appropriate ways of facilitating growth in the home setting. Both individual and group sessions are held to discuss progress and problems experienced by the parents. This model removes the pressure on parents of feeling that they are responsible for teaching their child, increases their knowledge, and provides demonstrations and models of appropriate interaction at each child's level. As well, it provides peer and professional support during the child's year long involvement in the programme.

The Hanen Early Language Parent Programme has much in common with the ELIP (Manolson, 1977, 1983). The programme was developed to overcome the inadequacy of the speech pathologist's traditional clinical role in providing services to the language delayed child. Realization that normal patterns of communicative interaction frequently do not occur when a delayed child presents confusing cues and reduced responsiveness to parents (Laskey and Allen, 1977), led to the establishment of a programme which aims at providing parents with the skills and experience to stimulate language growth at the prelinguistic and linguistic levels in the natural home environment. Informal teaching focuses on facilitating interaction by responsiveness to the child, following his or her lead in play, encouraging child participation, and ensuring the child has opportunity for turn-taking. It also emphasizes increasing semantically contingent strategies such as initiating, expanding, modelling, parallel talk and reducing the number of closed questions and demands. All of these strategies are well aligned with the responsiveness theory of language facilitation. The formal part of the programme follows the structured and semi-structured procedures outlined in the ELIP (MacDonald *et al.*, 1974). Parents are videotaped in the home setting and feedback is provided in group discussions on the faciliatory quality of the interaction. Efficacy data have demonstrated improvement in children's communication skills and significant change in the teaching skills and attitudes of the parents (Manolson, 1977). More recent research from this programme (Girolametta, 1985) has focused on the extent to which it has been effective in increasing conversational skills, and turn-taking behaviour in particular.

Turn-taking skills have been seen as a prerequisite to language development, a process which the child must learn, and the process through which learning is facilitated (Wells, 1980). Evidence that developmentally delayed children experience difficulty in turn-taking, topic-initiating and topic-continuing behaviours, and thus fail to receive feedback from mothers in the same manner as normal language learning children do, has been presented by Jones (1980) and Cunningham *et al.* (1981). The latter study aimed to investigate the structural aspects of the behaviour, such as length, size and quantity of turns, topical aspects such as the establishment of joint focus and the development of topic across speaking turns, as well as the children's communication skills. The twelve week programme included suggestions to parents regarding reducing the number of topics they initiated, increasing their responsiveness to their children's communicative attempts, keeping the conversation going for longer sequences on a topic, and increasing child initiations. Both experimental and control groups involved a mixture of Down's and other developmentally delayed children. At post-test, experimental mothers demonstrated an increase in turn-taking, topic maintenance and overall responsiveness to the child. Children initiated more topics, took part in longer turn sequences and displayed a significant increase in turns containing words, with a decrease in non-verbal turns. Parents were satisfactorily following the child's lead and providing feedback on the child's topic, thus facilitating the use of words in conversational contexts as the children maintained their turn-taking in longer sequences. No change in child language level was evident when measured on the SICD. This reflects the problems in measuring change in language skills over relatively short periods of time for mentally retarded children. A further comment by Girolametta (1985) on the population in his study relates to the wide range of developmental levels, and he emphasized the necessity of separating effects for children at different levels, a problem faced by all researchers using populations of mixed developmental level.

McConkey (1980) has long argued for implementation in the classroom of research findings on the early language development of mentally handicapped children, and has been actively involved in training teachers, preschool teachers, nurses, speech therapists and other para-professionals. At the same time, he has argued that the central role in facilitating early language in delayed children is that of the parent, and that the role of professionals is to increase the parents' knowledge about how this early learning takes place to enable them to help their child more effectively (McConkey, 1979). McConkey's work and programmes have differed from others in his emphasis on the relationship between cognitive growth and linguistic development. He stresses the importance of play in child learning and suggests that the different levels of play provide the experiences which the child needs in order to become familiar with the objects and actions and relations in his or her environment.

Until he or she reaches the representational stage of play, where a shoe box can 'become' a bed, the child is unable, cognitively, to deal with the idea of a particular set of sounds, namely a word, representing an object or action. The information provided to parents about the importance of involving children in play, and observing the level of play, allows the parent to understand the reason for the delay in vocal language. The emphasis on careful observation which, in his most recent programme (McConkey and Price, 1986), is extended to cover the child's earliest non-verbal communications, provides the parent with an orientation to the child which is almost inevitably responsive, and which should facilitate interactions at all stages of language learning. An understanding of the process by which language is acquired allows the parent to accept the notion that he or she cannot teach the child language, but can provide the optimal language learning environment by observing and responding to every communicative attempt the child makes, by involving the child in increasingly complex joint play activities, which enable him or her to learn about the world and, finally, to talk about it.

The range of programmes currently in operation, their responsiveness to changing theoretical and empirical perspectives, and the increasing awareness amongst parents and professionals that young developmentally delayed children can be helped to communicate effectively are all causes for satisfaction and optimism. Certainly programmes need to be more widely available, and many research issues remain unclarified, complicating the task of those involved in intervention, but immense progress has been made in the last decade, and there is no reason to believe that this will not continue into the 1990s.

The final section will review what we know about early language intervention and attempt to establish guidelines for future developments.

Some Guidelines for Future Early Language Intervention Programmes

Tremendous progress has been made in the last decade in one of the most important and difficult skill areas. Carefully designed intervention procedures, informed by current theory and research, are now providing services to thousands of children who may not succeed in acquiring adequate communication skills unless they receive special help. This includes children with specific language delay and disorders as well as children who are generally developmentally delayed. Advances are being made with programmes for severely handicapped populations (MacDonald, 1985; McLean and Snyder-McLean, 1987). To ensure continued progress we need to make certain that all professionals working with young language delayed children have comprehensive and detailed knowledge about the process and procedures of early language acquisition and intervention, understand the theoretical formulations which underpin them, and are in touch with current research efforts which must inform future developments in the field. Knowledge and support must be available to all parents who seek help for their children in developing their early language skills. If these conditions are met, then we can look forward to an increasingly vocal population of young people, able to express their needs and emotions, and to communicate satisfactorily with those around them.

Based on current theory and research evidence it seems probable that modifications to current programmes, and that programmes developed in the future will be less structured rather than more so. Programmes will be organized so that the goals are meaningful to the child in his or her attempts to communicate, and that they will be incorporated into the natural, everyday life of the child. Every opportunity for communication will be used, rather than setting aside particular times and places for 'teaching' language. The general theoretical framework which has the caregiver's interactions with the child as its central tenet implies that 'intervention' takes place whenever the child is interacting in a meaningful, communicative manner with any significant person, child or adult, in his or her natural environment. The role of intervention will be to ensure that the significant people in the child's life understand the process by means of which the child acquires language skills, and the crucial role that they can play in making the child's task easier. Parents and significant others may need to be taught to observe the child's earliest communicative attempts from infancy, to respond to them and to engage the child in meaningful, shared activity whenever possible in the course of the child's daily routines in his or her natural environment. Individual variation in parental knowledge and receptivity, and the extent of the child's handicapping condition, will determine how much 'teaching' and demonstration are required to ensure that the interactions are positive and provide the child with the experiences and framework which he or she requires for growth. The detailed steps in an intervention programme must be flexible enough to cater to individual differences and a variety of settings.

CONCLUSIONS

The general tenor of the material reviewed in this chapter suggests the following broad principles for facilitating language development through enhancing the quality of parent–child interaction:

1. Language cannot be 'taught', but a facilitating environment can be provided. This can best be achieved by ensuring that the caregivers, and all significant people in the child's life, in all the environmental settings in which the child spends his or her time, understand the process of language acquisition and the important role which can be played by everyone who interacts with the child. This applies to preschool teachers as well as parents, to siblings, grandparents and any other significant people who play a major role in the child's daily routine. The level of knowledge required can be varied according to the situation — but even a young sibling can learn to respond to any communicative attempts made by the child, and to follow his or her lead in any game or activity in which they may be jointly involved.

2. Communication must be 'environmental' - based on the child's needs and interests in everyday life situations. Where the situation is unfamiliar, the child relies upon interaction with his or her caregiver to make the situation meaningful.

3. The child learns to communicate through being involved in conversation with a mature language user, a responsive, caring adult who understands the need for the interaction to be child-centred, and who provides the necessary support to allow the child to use his or her language at whatever level he or she is capable. This sensitive interaction enables the child to reach new levels of achievement in partnership, which can later be achieved unaided an example of Bygotsky's 'zone of proximal development', referred to earlier in the chapter.

4. The significant interacting adult need not be the parent in all cases and at all times, although it inevitably is in the early stages of infancy. Intervention with toddlers and preschoolers can follow different models.

   a) Parents can be trained to take the main facilitation role with their own children, by attending a programme jointly with their child, being involved in the assessment, targeting appropriate goals, and 'working' with their child within the framework of the programme, and in all the everyday situations of the child's natural life. This approach has been used by MacDonald *et al.* (1974), Manolson (1977) and Bochner *et al.* (1982), and has proved very successful with some dyads, but may be too stressful for some parents who are faced with many extra problems related to raising a child who has a handicapping condition.

   b) Parent involvement can be through observation and discussion with staff attached to a preschool programme in which the children are enrolled in group sessions with individual programming. Parents are able to observe their children in interaction with the teachers and aides in the programme, to learn about the stages of language development, and how to follow the child's lead and engage the child in conversational interaction at the appropriate level. This knowledge is put into practice whenever the parents are interacting with their children in the course of their daily lives. This programme model provides support to parents, and indirect instruction, discussion and advice about progress and problems which arise in the home situation. This model is exemplified in the more recent work at the Macquarie University Special Education Centre (Bochner, 1987), where the effect of interactions in different classroom context, and with other children is being explored.

5. Programme style and steps must be flexible enough to cater for individual differences in both parents and children in terms of ability, problems, personality and learning styles. If the principles of early language acquisition are understood, then they can be applied in any setting by any person who is closely involved with the language-learning child. A variety of strategies must be available to help parents involve really difficult children in joint activities long enough for the child to learn turn-taking skills — the development of routine activities, nursery rhymes, action songs and finger plays, games which can be repeated over and over and which involve the passive child physically. Lists of suitable activities are becoming more frequent in materials developed by various language programmes (Bochner *et al.*, 1982; McConkey and Price, 1986).

6. Intervention should be available from the earliest stages of infancy to assist parents to recognize early, but inadequate, communicative attempts made by their child, and to learn how to be responsive in the face of unresponsive and difficult child behaviour. This may help to prevent the intractable problems faced in intervention when the parent and child have established a long-term confrontational interaction pattern. Many 'difficult' dyads would have benefitted from assistance in establishing reciprocity in infancy, where the problem has its roots.

7. Early intervention programmes concerned with communication and language acquisition need to be continually informed by and responsive to current research findings. Janko and Bricker (1987) discuss the problems associated with this. They refer to the huge investment in time and energy which is

required to establish a programme, and that major changes to the structure and operation are both costly and disruptive and cannot be undertaken lightly. This accounts for the excessive time lag which exists very often between the publication of research findings which have significance and their incorporation into language intervention practice. A further problem is trying to identify those findings which have significance and are of long lasting value, amongst the many controversial findings reported, and to ensure that the research base was wide and sound, and relevant to the population with whom the programme is dealing. The dilemma lies in resisting change and pursuing procedures which may not be as effective as modified practices based on current knowledge would be, on the one hand, and, on the other, adopting isolated findings without a full understanding of their implications in terms of the total theoretical framework. This problem can be solved by evaluating new findings with the wisdom of experience, and by maintaining as much flexibility in both planning and procedures as is possible. Not to incorporate important new findings condemns our children to a less than optimal learning environment, which in turn retards their progress in the already difficult task of acquiring early language and communication skills.

To summarize, we recommend that early intervention programmes should take into account the following points with regard to enhancing language development:

a) Language cannot be taught — but a facilitating environment can be provided by all those who interact with the child.

b) Communication must be based on the child's needs and interests in everyday life situations.

c) The child learns to communicate through conversation with a responsive, caring adult.

d) A variety of ways of training parents to facilitate their child's language and communication skills can be used.

e) Early intervention programmes must be flexible enough to cater for individual differences in both children and adults.

f) Intervention programmes should be available from the earliest stages of infancy.

g) Early intervention programmes should be continually informed by and responsive to current research findings on communication and language acquisition.

REFERENCES

Anastasiou, N.J. (1981) 'Early Childhood Education for the Handicapped in the 1980s: Recommendations,' *Exceptional Children, 47,* 4, 276–282.

Bellinger, D. (1980) 'Consistency in the Pattern of Change in Mothers Speech: Some Discriminant Analyses,' *Journal of Child Language, 7,* 469–487.

Bloom, B. (1973) *One Word at a Time: The Use of Single Word Utterances Before Syntax,* Mouton, The Hague.

Bochner, S. (1987) 'Preparation for Preschool: Report on a Programme for Language-Delayed 3 Year Olds,' *Paper presented at a Conference "Growing into a Modern World",* Centre for Child Research, University of Trondheim, Norway, June.

Bochner, S., Price, P. and Salamon, L. (1982) *Learning to Talk,* Special Education Centre, Macquarie University, Sydney.

Bochner, S., Price, P., Salamon, L., and Richardson, J. (1986) 'Language Intervention in the Pre-school Using a Parent Group Training Model,' *Australian Journal of Communication Disorders* 14, 2, 55–64.

Bower, T.G.R. (1971) *Human Development,* W.H. Freeman, San Francisco.

Bower, T.G.R. (1974) *Development in Infancy,* W.H. Freeman, San Francisco

Bower, T.G.R. and Wishart, J.G. (1979) 'Towards a Unitary theory of development,' in E.B. Thoman (ed.), *Origins of the Infant's Social Responsiveness.*

Bowerman, M. (1973) *Early Syntactic Development: A Cross-Linguistic Study with Special Reference to Finnish,* Cambridge, Mass.

Braine, M. (1963) 'The Ontogeny of English Phrase Structure. The First Phrase,' *Language, 39*, 1–13.

Bricker, D. and Carlson, L. (1980) 'An Intervention Approach for Communicatively Handicapped Infant's and Young Children,' *New Directions for Exceptional Children, 2.*

Bronson, G. (1978) 'Aversive Reactions to Strangers: A Dual Process Interpretation,' *Child Development, 49*, 495–499.

Brooks, J. and Lewis, M. (1976) 'Infants' Responses to Strangers: Midget, Adult and Child,' *Child Development, 47*, 323–332.

Bruner, J. (1977) 'Early Social Interaction and Language Interaction,' in H.R. Schaffer (ed.), *Studies in Mother–Infant Interaction*, Academic Press, New York.

Cairns, S., Pieterse, M., Treloar, R. and Gross, M. (1982) *T.E.L.L.: A Program for Developing Early Communication Skills*, Macquarie University, Down's Syndrome Program, Macquarie University.

Chomsky, N. (1957) *Syntactic Structures*, Mouton, The Hague.

Chomsky, N. (1965) *Aspects of a Theory of Syntax*, MIT Press, Cambridge, Mass.

Conti-Ramsden, G. (1985) 'Mothers in Dialogue with Language-Impaired Children,' *Topics in Language Disorders, 5*, 58–68.

Cross T. (1981) 'The Linguistic Experience of Slow Learners,' in A.R. Nesdale (ed.), *Advances in Child Development*, Cambridge University, Cambridge.

Cunningham, C., Reuler, E., Blackwell, and Deck, J. (1981) 'Behavioural and linguistic developments in the interactions of normal and retarded children with their mothers,' *Child Development, 52*, 62–70.

Eimas, P.D. and Tartter, V.C. (1979) 'The Development of Speech Perception,' in H.W. Reese and L.P. Lipsett (eds), *Advances in Child Development and Behaviour (Vol. 13)*, Academic Press, New York.

Fagan, J. (1976) 'Infants' Recognition of the Invariant Features of Faces,' *Child Development, 47*, 627–638.

Garcia, Eugene E. and de Haven, Everett D. (1974). 'Use of Operant Techniques in the Establishment and Genralization of Language: A Review and Analysis,' *American Journal of Mental Deficiency, 79*, 2, 169–178.

Girolametta, L. (1985) 'Hanen Early Language Parent Program,' *Paper presented to the Canadian Speech and Hearing Association Annual Convention.*

Halliday, M.A.K. (1975) *Learning How to Mean: Explorations in the Development of Language*, Edward Arnold, London.

Hart, B. and Risley, T. (1974) 'Using Preschool Materials to Modify the Language of Disadvantaged Children,' *Journal of Applied Behaviour Analysis*, 7, 243–256.

Hart, B. and Rogers-Warren, A. (1978) 'A Milieu Approach to Teaching Language,' in R.L. Shiefelbusch (ed.), *Language Intervention Strategies*, University Park Press, Baltimore.

Hayden, A. and Dimitriev, V. (1975) 'The Multidisciplinary Preschool Program of Down's Syndrome Children at the University of Washington Model Preschool Center,' in B. Friedlander, G. Sterrit and G. Kirk (eds), *Exceptional Infant, Vol. 3*, Brunner Mazel, New York.

Heber. R. and Garber, H. (1975) 'The Milwaukee Project: A Study of the Use of Family Intervention to Prevent Cultural-Familial Mental Retardation,' in B. Friedlander, G. Sterrit and G. Kirk (eds), *Exceptional Infant, Vol. 3*, Brunner Mazel, New York.

Hedrick. D.L., Prather, E.M. and Tobin, A.R. (1965) Sequenced Inventory of Communication Development, University of Seattle Press, Seattle.

Horstmeier, D.S. and MacDonald, J.D. (1975) *Ready, Set, Go: Talk To Me: Individualized Programs for Use in Therapy, Home and Classroom*, Charles E. Merrill, Ohio.

Jones, O. (1980) 'Prelinguistic Communication Skills in Down's Syndrome and Normal Infants,' in T. Fields (ed.), *High-Risk Infants and Children*, Academic Press, New York.

Laskey, E. and Allen, D. (1977) 'The Effects of Parent Training Programs on the Mother's Language Patterns Directed to Her TMR Child,' *Paper presented to the American Speech and Hearing Association, Chicago*.

Lennenberg, E. (1967) *Biological Foundations of Language*, Wiley, New York.

MacDonald, J. (1985) 'Language Through Conversation: A Model for Interventions with Language-Delayed Persons,' in S.F. Warren and A.K. Rogers-Warren (eds), *Teaching Functional Language*, Pro-Ed, Austin.

MacDonald, J., Blott, U., Gordon, K., Spiegel, B. and Hartmann, M. (1974) 'An Experimental Parent-Assisted Treatment Program for Pre-School Language-Delayed Persons,' *Journal of Speech and Hearing Disorders*, 39, 4, 395–414.

Manolson, H. (1977) Parents as language teachers. *Paper presented to the Annual Convention of the Canadian Speech and Hearing Association*.

Manolson, A. (1983) *It Takes Two To Talk*, Hanen Early Language Resource Centre, Toronto.

McConkey, R. (1979) 'Reinstating Parental Involvement in the Development of Communication Skills,' *Child: Care, Health and Development, 5,* 17–27.

McConkey, R. (1980) 'Implementation in the Classroom of Research Findings on the Early Language Development of Mentally Handicapped Children,' *First Language, 1,* 63–77.

McConkey, R. and Price, P. (1986) *Let's Talk,* Souvenir Press, London.

McLean, J. and Snyder-McLean, L. (1978) *A Transactional Approach to Early Language Training,* Merrill, Columbus, Ohio.

McLean, J. and Snyder-McLean (1987) 'Form and Function of Communicative Behaviour Among Persons with Severe Developmental Disabilities,' *Australia and New Zealand Journal of Developmental Disabilities, 13,* 2, 83–98.

McNeill, D. (1970) *The Acquisition of Language,* Harper and Row, New York.

Mitchell, D.R. (1987) 'Parents' Interactions with Their Developmental Disabled or At-Risk Infants: A Focus for Intervention,' *Australia and New Zealand Journal of Developmental Disabilities, 13,* 2, 73–82.

Moerk, E.L. (1976) 'Processes of Language Teaching and Training in the Interactions of Mother–Child Dyads,' *Child Development, 47,* 1064–1078.

Mowrer, O.H. (1954) 'The Psychologist Looks at Language,' *American Psychologist, 9,* 660–694.

Mowrer, O.H. (1958) 'Hearing and Speaking: An Analysis of Language Learning,' *Journal of Speech and Hearing Disability, 23,* 143–151.

Nelson, K. (1973) 'Structure and Strategy in Learning to Talk,' *Monograph of the Society for Research in Child Development, 38,* (Nos 1, 2, Serial No. 149).

Piaget, J. (1978) *The Development of Thought: Equilibration of Cognitive Structures,* Blackwell, Oxford.

Price, P. (1988) 'Language Intervention and Mother–Child Interaction' in M. Bevridge, G. Conti-Ramsden, and I. Leuder (eds), *Language and Communication in Mentally Handicapped People,* Chapman and Hall, London.

Price, P. and Bochner, S. (1984) 'Report of an Early Environmental Language Intervention Program,' *Australia and New Zealand Journal of Developmental Disabilities, 10,* 4, 217–228.

Sameroff, A. (1975) 'Early Influences on Development: Fact or Fancy?,' *Merrill-Palmer Quarterly, 21,* 267–294.

Shearer, D. and Shearer, M. (1976) 'The Portage Project: A Model for Early Childhood Intervention,' in T. Tjossem (ed.), *Intervention Strategies for High Risk Infants and Young Children,* University Park Press, Baltimore.

Skinner, B.F. (1957) *Verbal Behaviour*, Appleton-Century Crofts, New York.

Snow, C., Perlmann, R. and Nathan, D. (1985) *Why Routines are Different: Toward a Multiple-Factors Model of the Relation Between Input and Language Acquisition*, Harvard University, Cambridge.

Snyder, L. and McLean, J. (1976) 'Deficient Acquisition Strategies: A Proposed Conceptual Framework for Analyzing Severe Language Deficiency,' *American Journal of Mental Deficiency, 81*, 4, 338–349.

Vygotsky, L.S. (1962) *Thought and Language*, (L.E. Haufman and G. Vakar, translation), M.I.T. Press, Cambridge, Mass.

Wells, G. (1980) 'Adjustments in Adult–Child Conversation: Some Effects of Interaction' in H. Giles, P. Robinson, and P. Smith (eds), *Language*, Pergamon Press, Oxford, pp. 41–48.

Wells, G. (1981) *Learning Through Interaction*, Cambridge University Press, London.

Wells, G. (1985) *Language Development in the Pre-School Years*, Cambridge University Press, Cambridge.

Werner, H. and Kaplan, B. (1964) *Symbol Formation*, Wiley, New York.

10 EDUCATION AND TRAINING OF EARLY INTERVENTION PROGRAMME PERSONNEL

Roy V. Ferguson and Dana Brynelsen

INTRODUCTION

The past two decades have been a period of rapid growth in early intervention programmes for disabled and at-risk infants and young children and their families. One of the primary factors which seems to be driving this growth is the concept of continuity between early experience and later development. This relationship, although questioned by some, is the foundation upon which most early intervention and prevention programmes are predicated. Also, due to advances in medical science, greater numbers of at-risk infants are now surviving, resulting in the subsequent need for programmes designed to maximize the developmental potential of these infants. Other factors, such as a shift from institutional to community-based care and changing legislative mandates for disabled and at-risk infants and young children, are also contributing to the growth of early intervention programmes. The early intervention field is evolving and will continue to evolve as new situations, such as children with AIDS, present themselves.

While early intervention services are growing, it would appear that the preparation of personnel for these programmes has not kept pace. Katz (1984) notes that the majority of persons teaching children under the age of five years have no preservice preparation and only sporadic and limited inservice preparation. This situation exists in all countries and is the result of a combination of complex historical, political and economic forces (Goodnow and Burns, 1984). Certainly, it has a direct influence on the quality of the services being provided since the competence and attitudes of personnel are major determinants of programme effectiveness. It is difficult to provide quality care in programmes staffed by persons not well prepared to work with children below the age of three years, particularly when specific disabilities are involved.

Compounding the problem of lack of adequately prepared personnel is the limited literature relating to the education and training of early intervention personnel. Bricker and Slentz (1985) note, in regards to personnel preparation, 'a surprisingly sparse information base in comparison to the breadth and depth of publications available relevant to other aspects of early intervention' (p.22). There is an urgent need for the development of principles and guidelines specifically for the preparation of early intervention programme personnel so that some degree of standardization and coordination of the field can be achieved. This must be done in conjunction with careful research to examine the many issues and factors involved in providing effective education and training.

A reciprocal relationship exists between the practitioner role and professional preparation. The existing practitioner role influences the development of core curriculum in educational preparation programmes which, in turn, shape and consolidate the definition of the role and function of subsequent early intervention personnel. The remainder of this chapter will examine some of the key aspects of the practitioner role and their relationship to pre-service and inservice preparation programmes.

PRACTITIONER ROLE

The rapid expansion of early intervention programmes over the past two decades has resulted in a situation where practitioner roles and functions have been in a state of flux. There appears, however, to be an evolution towards greater similarity in philosophy, policy and practice in these programmes within and across countries, which should lead to a greater degree of standardization in practitioner roles (Mitchell, Brynelsen and Holm, 1988; Brown in this volume). In fact, this is already happening through the work of Bricker (1986), in the United States, who has clearly outlined five major early intervention programme personnel roles: conceptualizer, synthesizer, instructor, evaluator and counsellor. Bricker describes the conceptualizer as approaching teaching from a broad conceptual base while the synthesizer seeks and coordinates input from various professionals who are involved in the intervention. An instructor provides information and models instructional approaches for parents and paraprofessionals while an evaluator designs and implements strategies for determining programme effectiveness. Lastly, the counsellor listens, questions, provides feedback and assists families in problem solving.

Many of the major roles outlined above are implicit in the functioning of staff involved in early intervention programmes in New Zealand, where government policy emphasizes that all programmes should be designed to reflect the principles of parental involvement, a problem solving orientation and interdisciplinary cooperation (Brown, 1987). In Canada, Brynelsen and Cummings (1987) describe the functioning of infant development programmes as encompassing knowledge, skills and personal characteristics. The knowledge base would include: normal growth and development; learning theories; understanding the impact of a delay or handicap on child and family; assessment, programme planning and evaluation; roles of other professionals; and community resources. Communication, counselling and organizational skills are important to good clinical functioning. Personal characteristics considered important include: acceptance and respect for handicapped children and families, a belief in the ability of persons to change and adapt, maturity, independence, flexibility, humour, and direct parenting experience.

A certain similarity seems evident in the practitioner role outlined across these three countries. However, the early intervention area is a relatively new one and there are a number of considerations that are influencing how the roles and functions of early intervention programme practitioners evolve. Three of these will be examined below.

Generalist versus Specialist

The nature of service delivery to infants and their families will be influenced in a major way, depending on whether the practitioners approach clinical interventions from a generalist or specialist perspective. A specialist focus would result in the practitioner functioning in a manner similar to other, allied specialist roles such as psychology, occupational therapy, physiotherapy or speech therapy. A specialized knowledge about infancy and infant development and education would constitute the specific expertise brought to the programme. A generalist focus would create a practitioner who functions in a variety of roles including assessment, intervention and evaluation, and who has knowledge and skills in areas such as growth and development, principles of learning, programme planning, interpersonal communications, team collaboration, research/evaluation, and parental counselling. A major function of the generalist practitioner role would be to coordinate the therapeutic input from allied professionals so as to create an integrated programme for the infant and family.

There are situations in which either the specialist or generalist role has relative advantages. For example, working with specific populations such as people with visual or hearing impairments requires some specialized knowledge and skills. Consequently, specialized programmes tend to develop in large urban areas where there are greater numbers of individuals and families with similar specific needs and where there is a sufficient university/professional base to provide the necessary support to these programmes. Alternatively, programmes serving broader or mixed populations require practitioners who can function as generalists. In a review of early intervention programmes in the United States Bricker, Bailey and Bruder (1984) found that the majority were using their personnel as generalists who were responsible for the coordination of input from various professional specialists. A similar trend towards a generalist orientation in child and youth care practitioners in Canada is noted by Ferguson and Anglin (1985) and in New Zealand by Hornby and Murray (1987) who note a shift towards a generic rather than categorical role for special educators.

Multidisciplinary, Interdisciplinary and Transdisciplinary Roles

Early intervention programmes usually comprise of a collection of professionals from different disciplines collectively working towards common treatment goals for the children and families involved. The manner in which these professionals approach collaboration can be grouped into three general categories or levels. The first level of functioning is the multidisciplinary team in which the professionals meet as a group for planning purposes, but each discipline remains independent and is affected very little by the contributions of other team members. The next level is the interdisciplinary team which Fordyce (1982) suggested, 'differs from multidisciplinary in that the end product of the effort — the outcome — can only be accomplished by a truly interactive effort and contributions from the disciplines involved' (p.51). Next is the transdisciplinary team which has three characteristics (Lyon and Lyon, 1980): first, a joint team approach emphasizing collective problem solving around the client's needs; second, the expertise of individual team members is recognized and used to train other team members; and last, the roles and responsibilities are shared by more than one team member. Of course, there are unique problems to each of these team styles. For example, coordination of services to the client is difficult in a multidisciplinary team while group process problems are typical in an interdisciplinary team. In a transdisciplinary team, some members may experience difficulty in maintaining satisfactory professional identity in the practice of role exchange (Bailey, 1984).

The transdisciplinary model is considered to be the highest level of integrated team functioning (Meeth, 1978) and is most easily achieved by professionals with a generalist orientation since territoriality issues are less likely to be manifest. Interestingly, early intervention programmes located in rural areas often operate on a transdisciplinary team model. This is likely due to the fact that rural programmes are required to provide services to a wide range of disabilities with a smaller number of professional resources. Consequently, professionals in rural areas usually develop a generalist practice orientation which lends itself easily to a transdisciplinary service delivery model. Conversely, an interdisciplinary team model may be more appropriate in a programme comprising a larger number of professional specialists. It can also be highly effective, particularly if an emphasis is placed on collective problem-solving around the client's specific needs. In fact, many programme teams shift between multidisciplinary, interdisciplinary and transdisciplinary functioning in different circumstances relating to individual family needs.

Roles and functions of early intervention personnel are evolving towards a greater degree of uniformity. Within existing programmes, a preference is emerging for practitioners who are generalists skilled in interdisciplinary team functioning and able to coordinate input from various specialists.

Parent and Family Involvement

In recent years, professionals in the field of early childhood special education, realizing that the entire family is likely to influence and be influenced by the child's development, have become increasingly interested in the parents and families of handicapped children (Beckman and Burke, 1984; Cunningham and Davis, 1985; Mittler and McConachie, 1983; Hornby in this volume). A recognition has developed of the extent to which the family is influenced by the birth of a handicapped child (Beckman-Bell, 1981; Beckman, 1983) and the view has expanded from a focus primarily on mothers to one which includes fathers and siblings (Cansler, Martin, and Valand, 1975; Fewell, 1983). As a result, a growing emphasis on learning to work with parents and families is developing in professional preparation programmes for persons involved in early childhood education for the handicapped (Anastasiou, 1981; Tingey, Boyd, and Casto, 1987).

Legal mandates have also become more concerned with family involvment in early intervention programmes. For example, Bailey and Simeonsson (1988) point out that, while US Public Law 94-142 did not require that goals or services be specified for families, the subsequent passage of Public Law 99-457 did specify the need for individualized family service plans. Consequently, family assessments were necessary to identify individual family strengths and needs.

Further, programme approaches have tended to shift from a deficit to a proactive model of early intervention and this has a significant effect on the nature of family involvement in the programme. Where the deficit approach focuses the intervention on the remediation of deficits, the proactive approach focuses on strengthening families (Dunst, 1985). Interventions are aimed at empowering the families with knowledge and skills which give them access and control over resources necessary to meet family needs. Professionals encourage families to consider aspects of quality of life (Brown, 1988) when identifying their needs and establishing programme objectives. Families and professionals then work in a collaborative manner in pooling their respective strengths towards addressing mutually designed programme objectives. Working effectively with parents and families is, therefore, a particularly important part of the role of early intervention programme staff.

Now that key aspects of the early intervention practitioner role have been outlined, let us turn our attention to education and training programmes and how they are being designed to prepare personnel for the field.

PRESERVICE PROGRAMMES

Education and training programmes for early intervention personnel can be developed on a preservice or inservice basis. Preservice education and training is done through formal undergraduate or graduate programmes in post-secondary academic institutions where the student earns a certificate, diploma, or degree upon successful completion of the course of studies. Inservice activities are informal and ongoing in nature, typically occurring within the service delivery agency, and do not usually provide formal recognition of participant involvement.

The following will examine the structure, content and curriculum organization of preservice programmes.

Structure

It is important that practitioner preparation programmes focus specifically on the birth to three year old population and that this age group is seen as distinct from the older preschool population. This distinction is important because development during the birth to three and three to five age ranges is unique and different from other developmental intervals. Service delivery models are also different for these two age groups since older preschool children are usually involved in centre-based group programmes while infants and toddlers more typically are served at home on an individual basis. Further, the involvement of the family is more critical for children from birth to three as the primary focus in early intervention programmes is often on the caregiver.

Existing preservice preparation programmes are presently located in a variety of disciplinary or interdisciplinary domains including medical, educational and allied health (nursing, psychology, occupational therapy, speech therapy, etc.). While the location of the programme undoubtedly creates a particular emphasis in the curriculum content, no particular professional area is uniquely best suited for the development of these programmes. Appropriate curriculum content which spans all of the key professional areas is more important as a consideration than where the programme is located within an academic setting.

Similarly, within the service delivery system, early intervention programmes should not be seen as necessarily being situated within a particular type of service agency (e.g. health, education or social services) but, rather, should be located within the jurisdiction best suited to meet the unique needs and preferences of each community. In other words, no particular type of agency or jurisdiction is inherently better suited to the delivery of early intervention programmes in all situations. This view seems to be reflected in the recent Public Law 99-457 in the United States which is designed 'to develop and implement a statewide, comprehensive, coordinated, multidisciplinary, interagency programme of early intervention services for infants and toddlers with handicaps and their families'. (US Department of Education, 1987, p.44355). The responsibility for the implementation of this programme 'could be the department of education, health, mental health, or some other appropriate department of State government designated by the Governor' (p.44352).

Effective early intervention programmes are seen to be the product of interagency and interdisciplinary coordination. Since ownership of the area cannot be claimed by any individual discipline, preparation programmes for early intervention personnel will develop in a variety of different academic locations. Consequently, it is critical that a core curriculum be identified. A generic, core curriculum will provide a standardization in the preparation of early intervention personnel, regardless of the location of the education and training programme.

Curriculum Content

A common method in practitioner preparation has been to use a competency-based approach in which the students are required to demonstrate proficiency in a specified set of skills prior to programme completion. Common competency areas across many preparation programmes noted in the literature are ones such as child development, assessment, intervention planning and implementation, evaluation, teaching, family involvement, service coordination, administration, environmental manipulation, ecological perspective, interdisciplinary team functioning and programme evaluation (Bricker andIacino, 1977; Fewell, 1983; Geik, Gilkerson and Sponseller, 1982; Mallory, 1983; Miller, 1977). In response to the scattered and limited information available on training programme content and structure, Bricker and Slentz (1985) conducted a national survey in the United States. They found that there were seven general competency areas consistently noted across the programmes which were surveyed.

These common areas are listed below as well as some of the content material which might be included in each of them, are listed below.

Knowledge of Typical (normal) Child Development
- prenatal, perinatal, infant and child development
- cognitive, physical/motor, perceptual, social and language
- developmental influences, environmental interactions
- developmental assessment.

Knowledge of Atypical (abnormal) Child Development
- prenatal and postnatal developmental disruptions
- developmental disabilities

Education and Training of Personnel

Assessment (developmental and behavioural) Skills
- psychometric principles (scales, reliability, validity)
- instrumentation
- behavioural observation.

Programme Development Skills
- existing programme resources
- individual, small and large group programme development
- goal statements relating to assessment data
- programme planning
- implementation
- evaluation
- follow-up.

Intervention (teaching) Strategies
- small and large group intervention/instruction/activity
- environmental modification
- programme coordination
- personnel supervision.

Data Dollection and Individual Programme Monitoring Skills
- design and manage data management systems
- interdisciplinarity, allied professionals
- programme evaluation
- professional conduct
- service delivery networks
- legislation
- advocacy

Parent Training and Family Involvement Skills
- family systems
- effects of handicaps on families
- family adaptive mechanisms
- parents as partners in programme
- parental consultation
- parental education

The authors of this survey note that while the above content areas emerged consistently across programmes, there were other competencies that were more idiosyncratic to individual programmes. This survey was instrumental in identifying the areas that were seen as common across programmes and constitutes an important planning base upon which to build curriculum in new programmes and to modify it in existing ones. The common areas identified can provide a guideline for a beginning generic core of content for all early intervention preparation programmes. These core courses would be augmented by various courses specific to the needs and resources of individual programmes.

Curriculum Organization

Academic programmes for the preparation of early intervention personnel should involve both education (a knowledge base) and training (applied skills). Further, an appropriate balance of theory and practice should exist across all levels of education and training (VanderVen, Mattingly and Morris, 1982).

In providing education and training for child and youth care professionals across a broad scope of service delivery settings (Ferguson, Denholm and Pence, 1987), the School of Child Care at the University of Victoria utilizes a curriculum model designed to facilitate integrated learning. It is built upon three, interactive structural pillars: knowledge, skills and self. The knowledge and skills elements are fairly traditional aspects of curriculum, although integrating them can often be a difficult task.

The third pillar (self) is somewhat more unique and addresses the individual aspects of the learner by considering factors such as values, attitudes, beliefs, learning style and experience. For example, a belief necessary to effectively working with parents in early intervention programmes is the proactive viewpoint mentioned earlier as important. In order to engage in collaborative goal-setting, a process by which parents and programme personnel jointly determine intervention goals (Bailey, 1987), the professional must believe that parents are partners in the intervention process and that the locus of decision making is with the family. Without the prerequisite foundation of values, attitudes and beliefs, it would be difficult, if not impossible, to establish in the learner the skills necessary for effective work with parents. Similarly, learners must understand their own values structures and how they relate to the values structures of the people with whom they will be working. In discussing values in the context of family therapy, Aponte (1985) points out that 'values frame the entire process of therapy' (p.323). The effectiveness of early intervention activities, then, is closely linked to the ability of the clinician in resolving value differences which may arise within the programme.

Another example of an aspect of the self component of curriculum design is learning style. Learning style can be described as a characteristic of an individual that interacts with instructional circumstances in such a way as to produce differential learning. If we accept this idea that all persons do not learn in the same way, it then becomes important for students to have an understanding of their learning style characteristics so that they can engineer educational conditions (e.g. amount of structure they prefer) under which they learn best. Similarly, an understanding of adult learning style characteristics prepares the professional to function more effectively in a teaching role with parents.

The self component of the curriculum functions in the manner of a 'lens,' focussing the knowledge and skill elements of curriculum content in a way which acknowledges the uniqueness of the individual learner (Figure 10.1).

Figure 10.1: Interactive curriculum organization.

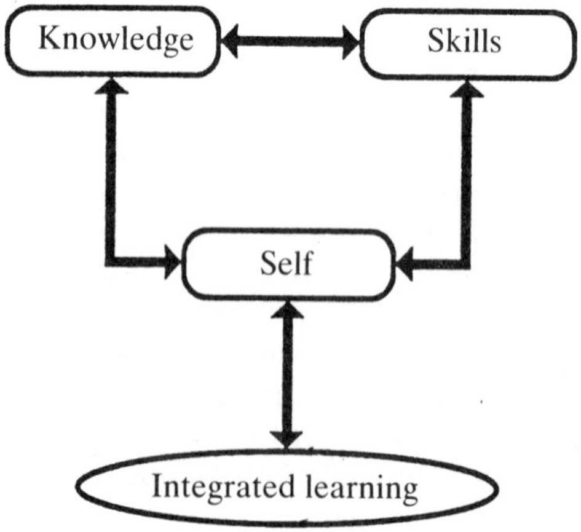

A consideration of individual aspects of the learner is particularly important for students who enter a training programme with considerable clinical experience, but is also central to the preparation of young and inexperienced students who are beginning to develop their professional attitude and value structure. It is suggested that good curriculum design for early intervention preparation programmes needs to consider the interaction of knowledge, skills and learner characteristics.

INSERVICE PROGRAMMES

Since the field is changing so rapidly and many of the present practitioners do not have formal preservice education, an important component of personnel preparation for early intervention programmes is inservice training. Inservice training can be defined as an ongoing and systematic mechanism of continued education and training to support the accomplishment of organizational and individual goals. Continuing education and ongoing training for programme personnel are key mechanisms for updating knowledge and skill levels, which, in turn, relate to better practice, improved morale, and lower programme staff turnover (Trohanis, 1985). Inservice programme models are diverse in regards to length, format, focus and content. Some are built upon a workshop format (Bloom, 1980), others on a summer institute model combining preservice and inservice components (Brynelsen, 1987), and some involve weekly activities over a number of months (Davis and Porter, 1981). The target of inservice programmes can be professionals, para-professionals, volunteers, or parents and the content varies according to the intended audience.

Parents are not only recipients in inservice programmes, but also have important contributions to make to them. Parents are increasingly being used to provide instruction to other parents and caregivers in early intervention programmes (Bricker, 1986). As they become more comfortable in their new partnership role developing in many programmes they will undoubtedly also be involved in the provision of inservice training to early intervention professionals. At this point the collaborative partnership will become complete.

Another approach which is not often considered is that of using formative conjoint evaluation as a vehicle for inservice training. Mitchell (1987) developed a Scale for Evaluating Early Intervention Programmes which was designed to assist in the development of quality early intervention programmes for developmentally disabled infants and young children and their families. Mitchell (also in the present volume) envisaged that his scale 'will primarily be employed in formative evaluation procedures in which evaluation is used as the basis for future planning by the management and staff of early intervention programmes' (p.38). Formative evaluation structures such as this provide programmes with useful feedback which staff and parents, during inservice sessions, can discuss and consider the implications for change.

Since most inservice programmes are designed to address specific needs, the differences across programmes are often greater than the similarities. This high degree of individualization is an important function of inservice training which preservice programmes are not able to perform because they must be more generic in their approach in order to establish a standardized foundation of education and training. Consequently, inservice training can exist independently or can be designed as an extension of preservice programmes. Often, preservice programme resources are called upon in the development of inservice training activities. This facilitates the linkage between the two mechanisms, but can place the rural early intervention programmes at a disadvantage because of the geographic distances involved. In response to this problem, and because students are often not able to attend a campus-based preservice programme, many post-secondary educational institutions are developing distance education offerings.

DISTANCE EDUCATION

A variety of different terminologies, including adult education, further studies, extramural studies, continuing education, extension learning and distance education are used interchangeably, although the latter seems to be the preferred term. Keegan (1980) lists the main elements of distance education as:

- the separation of teacher and learner which distinguishes it from face-to-face learning
- the influence of an educational organization that distinguishes it from private study
- the use of technical media, usually print, to unite teacher and learner and carry the educational content
- the provision of two way communications so that the student may benefit from, or even initiate, dialogue
- the possibility of occasional meetings for both didactic and socialization purposes (p.33).

In general, distance education involves the delivery of course material to adult learners who are remote from a centre, through the use of multiple delivery technologies and strategies.

There are a number of factors which are contributing to the recent growth of distance education. Rapidly changing technology and professional information mean that it is no longer possible to acquire a complete education at the beginning of a career. Lifelong learning and recurring education are universal needs which result in the increasing demand for continuing professional education. The growing role of women in the work force is also a key factor in expanding the need for distance education programmes, as is the increasing number of already well educated persons involved in mid-career change. It is also increasingly common for various occupational groups to require that their members be involved in a certain amount of continuing education each year in order to maintain practice credentials. Lastly, tighter economies have resulted in a restricted job market in which fewer persons are willing or able to leave their places of employment to seek out further education. Consequently, there has been a growing demand for more continuing education and inservice programmes which, in turn, lend themselves well to distance education format.

Colleges and universities, where preservice programmes are usually located, are often initially uncomfortable at the idea of learning occurring off campus and out of the classroom. There are also unique problems involved in the provision of distance education, such as professional socialization, library resources, student access to consultation/advising and transfer credit arrangements. However, with increasing experience at developing distance education offerings, most institutions find solutions to these problems and become comfortable with the idea of parallel on and off campus programmes and activities.

There are numerous economies and benefits in developing on and off campus offerings on a simultaneous basis and educational institutions with new or developing preservice early intervention preparation programmes would be well advised to consider distance education structures at the earliest possible point. Campbell (1984) cautions that 'there is reason to speculate that the university which neglects the continuing education of its graduates will have cause to regret it' (p. 23).

Distance education is developing rapidly in post-secondary educational institutions and is ideally suited to the preservice and inservice needs of early intervention personnel, many of whom require educational upgrading but are employed in programmes in rural areas. Distance education is also a mechanism which can provide education and training to new persons wishing to enter the early intervention field but not having easy access to a college or university.

SUMMARY AND CONCLUSIONS

Early intervention programmes for infants and toddlers with handicaps have been growing in number rapidly and, in view of new enabling legislation in some countries, will continue to develop at an even faster rate. Unfortunately, education and training for early intervention programme personnel has not kept pace, nor has research on professional development. Some degree of practitioner role standardization is beginning to develop in the field within and across countries and this is a vital step towards assisting the development of a generic, core curriculum in education and training programmes. A similar core curriculum in preservice practitioner preparation programmes, in turn, will help to consolidate the definition and standardization of the role and function of early intervention personnel. Further, inservice programmes need to be developed which are capable of meeting needs for continuing education. These inservice structures can function in a stand alone manner or be an extension of existing preservice programmes. Distance education has a major role to play in the provision of preservice and inservice education and training and should be developed on a coterminous basis with traditional educational programmes.

In an examination of the education and training of early intervention programme personnel the following were the key points considered:
1. The preparation of trained personnel has not kept pace with the growth of early intervention programmes in the past two decades.

2. Major roles of early intervention programme personnel include conceptualizer, synthesizer, instructor, evaluator and counsellor and are quite similar across programmes.

3. Within existing programmes a preference is noted for professionals who are generalist in their orientation, skilled in interdisciplinary team collaboration and able to work effectively with parents and families.

4. Preservice preparation programmes should be located in a variety of disciplinary locations within educational settings.

5. Seven generic core curriculum areas are noted which should be included in all early intervention personnel preparation programmes.

6. Curriculum content should be organized to include an interaction of knowledge, skills and learner characteristics.

7. Inservice structures can function independently or as an extension of preservice programmes in providing continuing education.

8. Distance education has been developing in colleges and universities as a mechanism to provide preservice and inservice education and training to persons not able to leave their employment or geographical area.

REFERENCES

Anastasiou, N. J. (1981) 'Early Childhood Education for the Handicapped in the 1980s: Recommendations,' *Exceptional Children*, 47, 276–282.
Aponte, H. J. (1985) 'The Negotiation of Values in Therapy,' *Family Process*, 24, 323–328.

Bailey, D. B. (1984) 'A Triaxial Model of the Interdisciplinary Team and Group Process,' *Exceptional Children, 1,* 17–25

Bailey, D. B. (1987) 'Collaborative Goal-setting with Families: Resolving Differences in Values and Priorities for Services,' *Topics in Early Childhood Special Education, 7,* 59–71.

Bailey, D.B. and Simeonsson, R.J. (1988) *Family Assessment in Early Intervention.* Merrill Publishing Co., Columbus, OH.

Beckman, P. J. (1983) 'The Influence of Selected Characteristics on Stress in Families of Handicapped Infants,' *American Journal of Mental Deficiency, 88,* 150–156.

Beckman, P. J. and Burke, P. J. (1984) 'Early- childhood Special Education: State of the Art,' *Topics in Early Childhood Special Education, 4,* 9–32.

Beckman-Bell, P. (1981) 'Child-Related Stress in Families of Handicapped Children,' *Topics in Early Childhood Special Education, 1,* 45–54.

Bloom, B. (1980) 'Preparing Paraprofessionals for Work with Families of Preschool Exceptional Children,' *Special Education in Canada, 56,* 7–8.

Bricker, D. (1986) *Early Education of At-risk and Handicapped Infants, Toddlers and Preschool Children,* Scott, Foresman and Co., Glenview, IL.

Bricker, D. and Iacino, R. (1977) 'Early Intervention with Severely/ Profoundly Handicapped Children,' in E. Sontag, J. Smith, and N. Certo (eds), *Educational Programming for the Severely and Profoundly Handicapped,* The Council for Exceptional Children, Reston, Virginia.

Bricker, D., Bailey, E., and Bruder, M. B. (1984) 'The Efficacy of Early Intervention and the Handicapped Infant,' in M. Wolraich and D. Routh (eds), *Advances in Developmental and Behavioral Pediatrics, Vol. 5,* JAI Press, Greenwich, CT.

Bricker, D. and Slentz, K. (1985) 'Personnel Preparation: Handicapped Infants,' *Manuscript developed for the Research Integration Project,* University of Pittsburgh.

Brown, D. (1987) 'Department of Education Early Intervention Programmes,' in D. Mitchell and C. Brown (eds), *Future Directions for Early Intervention,* Down's Association, Auckland, New Zealand.

Brown, R.I. (1988) 'Quality of Life and Rehabilitation: An Introduction,' in R. Brown (ed.) *Quality of Life for Handicapped People,* Croom Helm, London.

Brynelsen, D. (1987) 'Working Together: The British Columbia
	Approach to Early Intervention,' in D. Mitchell and C. Brown
	(eds), *Future Directions for Early Intervention*, Down's Associa-
	tion, Auckland, New Zealand.
Brynelsen, D. and Cummings, H. (1987) 'Infant Development Pro-
	grams: Early Intervention in Delayed Development,' in
	C. Denholm, R. Ferguson, and A. Pence (eds), *Professional Child
	And Youth Care: The Canadian Perspective*, University of British
	Columbia Press, Vancouver, B.C.
Campbell, D. D. (1984) *The New Majority: Adult Learners in the Uni-
	versity*, University of Alberta Press, Edmonton, AB.
Cansler, D. P., Martin, G. H., and Valand, M. C. (1975) *Working with
	Families*, Kaplan Press, Winston-Salem, NC.
Cunningham, C.C. and Davis, H. (1985) *Working with Parents*, Open
	University Press, Milton Keynes.
Davis, J. and Porter, M. (1981) 'An Inservice Training Program for
	Rural Area Professionals Concerned with Early Childhood
	Special Education,' in B. Smith-Dickson (ed.), *Making it Work in
	Rural Areas: Training, Recruiting*, and Retaining Personnel in
	Rural Areas, HCEEP Rural Network Monographs.
Dunst, C. J. (1985) 'Rethinking Early Intervention,' *Analysis and
	Intervention in Developmental Disabilities, Vol. 5*, Pergamon Press,
	New York.
'Early Intervention Program for Infants and Toddlers with Handi-
	caps' (1987) *Federal Register, 52*, 44352–44362.
Ferguson, R. V. and Anglin, J. P. (1985) 'The Child Care Profession:
	A Vision for the Future,' *Child Care Quarterly, 14*, 85–102.
Ferguson, R., Denholm, C. and Pence, A. (1987) 'An Overview of the
	Scope of Child Care in Canada,' in C. Denholm, R. Ferguson,
	and A. Pence (eds), *Professional Child and Youth Care: The Cana-
	dian Perspective*, University of British Columbia Press, Vancou-
	ver, B.C.
Fewell, R.R. (1983a) 'The Team Approach to Infant Education,' in
	S. Garwood and R.R. Fewell (eds), *Educating Handicapped In-
	fants: Issues in Development and Intervention*, Aspen, Rockville,
	MD.
Fewell, R. R. (1983b) 'Assessing Handicapped Infants,' in S. G. Gar-
	wood and R. R. Fewell (eds.), *Educating Handicapped Infants:
	Issues in Development and Intervention*, Aspen, Rockville, MD.
Fordyce, W. E. (1982) 'Interdisciplinary Process: Implications for
	Rehabilitation Psychology,' *Rehabilitation Psychology, 27*, 5–11.

Geik, I., Gilkerson, L., and Sponseller, D. (1982) 'An Early Interven-
    tion Training Model,' *Journal for the Division of Early Childhood, 5,*
    42–52.
Goodnow, J. and Burns, A. (1984) 'Factors Affecting Policies in Early
    Childhood Education: An Australian Case,' in L. G. Katz,
    P. J. Wagemaker, and K. Steiner (eds), *Current Topics in Early
    Childhood Education, Vol. 5,* Ablex Publishing Corporation,
    Norwood, New Jersey.
Hornby, G. and Murray, R. (1987) 'Preparation of Professionals for
    Special Education,' in D. R. Mitchell and N. N. Singh (eds), *Ex-
    ceptional Children in New Zealand,* Dunmore Press, Palmerston
    North, New Zealand.
Katz, L. G. (1984) 'The Education of Preprimary Teachers,' in
    L. G. Katz, P. J. Wagemaker, and K. Steiner (eds), *Current Topics
    in Early Childhood Education, Vol. 5,* Ablex Publishing Corpora-
    tion, Norwood, New Jersey.
Keegan, D. J. (1980) 'On Defining Distance Education,' *Distance
    Education, 1,* 13–36.
Lyon, S. and Lyon, G. (1980) 'Team Functioning and Staff Develop-
    ment: A Role Release Approach to Providing Integrated Educa-
    tional Services for Severely Handicapped Students,' *Journal of the
    Association for the Severely Handicapped, 5,* 250-263.
Mallory, B. (1983) 'The Preparation of Early Childhood Special
    Educators: A Model Program,' *Journal for the Division of Early
    Childhood, 7,* 32–40.
Meeth, R. L. (1978) 'Interdisciplinary Studies: A Matter of
    Definition,' *Change Magazine, 10,* 10–11.
Miller, P. (1977) 'Teacher Competencies in Early Education of the
    Handicapped,' in *Models for Training Teachers of Early Education
    for the Handicapped,* The Council for Exceptional Children,
    Reston, VA.
Mitchell, D. R. (1987) 'Evaluating Early Intervention Programmes for
    Young Children with Special Needs,' in D. Mitchell and
    C. Brown (eds), *Future Directions for Early Intervention, Down's
    Association,* Auckland, New Zealand.
Mitchell, D.R., Brynelsen, D. and Holm, M. (1988) 'Evaluating the
    Process of Early Intervention Programmes,' *Irish Journal of Psy-
    chology, 9,* 235–248.
Mittler, P. and McConachie, H. (1983) *Parents, Professionals and Men-
    tally Handicapped People,* Croom Helm, London.
Tingey, C., Boyd, R. D., and Casto, G. (1987) 'Parental Involvement in
    Early Intervention: Becoming a Parent-Plus,' *Early Child Devel-
    opment and Care, 27,* 91–105.

US Department of Education (1987) 'Early Intervention Program for Infants and Toddlers with Handicaps: Notice of Proposed Rulemaking,' *Federal Register, 52*, No. 222, November 18, Washington, D.C.

VanderVen, K., Mattingly, M., and Morris, M. (1982) 'Principles and Guidelines for Child Care Personnel Preparation Programs,' *Child Care Quarterly, 11*, 242–249.

11 EVALUATING PROGRAMME IMPACT: LEVELS OF CERTAINTY

Rune J. Simeonsson and Donald B. Bailey, Jr

INTRODUCTION

The number and variety of early intervention models and programmes for at-risk and handicapped infants and their families has increased dramatically in the last two decades. This increase can undoubtedly be attributed to the intrinsic appeal of early intervention which draws on concepts of stimulation and prevention from developmental psychology and medicine. The intrinsic nature of this appeal is grounded in the belief that early development is more plastic than later development and that intervention in this sensitive period is thus likely to have greater preventive or ameliorative effects than in other periods. This belief underlies most early intervention programmes and currently finds its expression in an array of programmes for handicapped and at-risk infants in hospitals, homes and child care facilities.

Evaluating the impact of early intervention as a means of preventing or ameliorating developmental disabilities in infants and young children, however, has been a long standing problem and its effectiveness continues to be debated (Casto and Mastropieri, 1986; Dunst and Snyder, 1987; Strain and Smith, 1987). The discrepancy between the popular acceptance of early intervention and equivocal efficacy evidence can be traced to three major limitations of early intervention research: (a) inadequate experimental rigour, (b) inadequate sample sizes and/or designs, and (c) inadequate and/or inappropriate outcome measures. These problems are difficult to resolve given practical as well as ethical expectations to provide a service that is widely perceived as needed if not essential. In recent years there has been a variety of efforts to address specific shortcomings of prior research studies. In addition to a number of conceptual (Meisels, 1985) as well as analytic (Ottenbacher, 1989; Shonkoff and Hauser-Cram, 1987) contributions, entire journal issues have been devoted to collections of studies designed to address one or more of earlier limitations of the literature (Dunst, 1985). Central to most of the studies were detailed descriptions of the subjects as well as the interventions that were provided for them. Taken collectively, these relatively well designed and well documented studies provide substantive evidence in support of the benefits of early intervention.

The acceptance of early intervention as a preventive and habilitative strategy will undoubtedly persist whether or not the status of impact evaluation improves. Given the fact that the arguments for early intervention may be as much logical and humanitarian as they are scientific, it may be unlikely that efficacy evidence *per se* is needed to justify its continued application. It is, in fact, ironic that efficacy evidence is seen as a prerequisite for the provision of intervention for infants and preschool children, whereas no similar prerequisite is demanded to legitimize intervention for school-aged children. The position taken here is that the premise for early intervention may be grounded in logical, theoretical, and humanitarian bases rather than exclusively empirical grounds. It is, in fact, reasonable to assume that early intervention for infants with handicaps would at this point continue to be endorsed even if a 'perfect' study yielded evidence 'proving' that it was not effective.

Given the current discrepancy between limited impact evidence and the universal belief in intervention efficacy, the focus of future evaluation efforts should be to improve the nature and form of intervention services through careful documentation rather than to 'prove' that intervention is effective in some general sense. Improvement of intervention as a focus for evaluation activities would address clinical as well as scientific concerns about accountability. While the concept of accountability can be interpreted in a number of ways, in its broadest sense it can be defined as the documentation that a needed intervention has been provided in an appropriate manner with the probability that at least some desired outcomes of been achieved. The issue of interest in clinical accountability is the extent to which services as perceived by both parents and professionals to be satisfactory and appropriate for child and family needs. Whether the concern is about a single child or a population, clinical accountability is concerned with documentation that an appropriate intervention was provided with a high probability that it was effective. Scientific accountability, on the other hand, can be defined as empirical evidence that interventions are causally linked to outcomes and furthermore, that the effects have the potential to be generalized across subjects and settings.

Addressing limitations of the early intervention efficacy literature, Meisels (1985) stressed that several major issues needed to be clarified before significant questions about the effectiveness of early intervention could be examined. These issues included clarification of the underlying model or rationale for early intervention; the nature of the intervention; the nature of outcome measurement; and the characteristics of the subjects of intervention. An evaluation perspective is needed that can provide a template by which each of the above issues can be clarified.

Viewed in this context, evaluation of early intervention will continue to be an essential activity, but a number of factors require that the focus and nature of evaluation change. Central to these is the growing complexity of the nature of early intervention services in which the focus of services has expanded to include the family in direct as well as indirect forms of support, consequently creating the need for a broader array of outcome variables. New conceptualizations of evaluation are needed which mirror the complexity and comprehensiveness of the changing status of early intervention. While experimental control and statistical rigour are often seen as desirable in evaluation, they may be neither attainable nor appropriate in many early intervention programmes. The nature of phenomena (infant and family behaviour) and the context in which it is approaches (clinical services) may not warrant the level of measurement and evaluation precision inherent in traditional experimental and analytic manipulations. Recognition of this issue suggests an approach to evaluation which takes varying levels of precision and proof into account. Such an approach requires that the following broad questions be addressed in the evaluation of programme impact:

1. What is the nature or level of intervention?
2. What is the level of precision of measurement?
3. To what degree is intervention implemented?
4. What is the level of proof of evaluation evidence?

The purpose of this chapter is to present a framework for evaluating impact in early intervention which addresses these broad questions. The framework specifies a hierarchical designation of levels of intervention (Simeonsson and Bailey, 1989) and an approach to evaluation issues defined by levels of certainty of evidence (Smith, 1981). To accomplish this purpose, a general rational for a dimensional approach to family involvement in early intervention will be complemented by a consideration of evaluation in terms of levels of certainty of measurement, implementation and evidence. The application of this framework in early intervention will be defined in terms of appropriate strategies and methods in the design and evaluation of intervention programmes.

LEVELS AND TYPES OF INTERVENTION

The growing literature on the evaluation of services for infants and preschoolers with handicaps and their families reveals that the term 'early intervention' is not a unitary construct expressed in one type of treatment. Rather it represents a complex interaction of direct and indirect services that vary significantly according to factors such as child needs, family preferences, professional skills and philosophy, and the resources available to specific service delivery systems. The following examples reflect the diversity of treatment contexts that could conceivably be considered to be early intervention:

— Programme A provides 'early intervention' for Alecia, who was born prematurely to a single, teenage mother who lives in an inner city housing project. A home-based interventionist makes weekly one-hour visits to the home. The mother is rarely there, as Alecia's grandmother and aunt share most of the child care responsibilities. The interventionist spends most of her time providing developmentally appropriate activities for Alecia and leaves suggestions for other stimulation activities that could be provided in between home visits.

—Programme B provides 'early intervention' for Manuel, who has Down's syndrome. Manuel attends a full day programme at a mainstreamed infant center staffed by an interdisciplinary team of specialists. Manuel's parents are very interested in the programme and have taken the initiative to form a parents' group that meets monthly.

These two cases provide one simple example of the considerable diversity of factors embedded within the early intervention construct. Any effort to answer the question 'Is early intervention effective?' must recognize that diversity consequently tailors the evaluation to the specific treatment provided.

Tailoring the evaluation question to the level and type of treatment provided is essential, but yet another variable must be brought into the equation: parental preferences for involvement and services. The importance of this information is exemplified in the following question: Which is more effective: an 'intense' treatment provided to a family that does not want it, or a 'mild' treatment provided for a family that desires it?

While the needs of the infant or young child continue to be the basis for access to early intervention services, the increased emphasis on the role of the family has resulted in greater diversity of involvement of child and family. From a historical perspective, the role of families in early intervention has broadened from one in which they were participants in the provision of services to their children to one in which they themselves assumed roles as clients and recipients of services (Simeonsson and Bailey, 1989).

Representatives of the participant role of families in early intervention services were instances in which a family member, typically the mother, becomes a member of the intervention team to extend its service objectives. Illustrative of parent involvement in service participation is the designation by Hanson (1985) as 'crucial members of the team...' (p. 40) is illustrative of parent involvement in service participation. Early intervention services in which families have assumed a client role however, are relatively more recent and models for such services are still evolving. Generally speaking, however, such services have focused on the provision of information, support and/or counselling for families relative to identified family needs. An example of this approach in early intervention is a study by Vadasy *et al.* (1986) in which fathers of handicapped children participated in father–child activities and were provided informational and support services suited to paternal needs.

The philosophical commitment to early intervention and its

enactment in services is increasingly evident in various forms across countries. The enactment and implementation of PL99-457, with its provision for an Individualized Family Service Plan (IFSP) is likely to increase the client role of the family in early intervention services. As such services expand and become more formalized, a framework is needed to conceptualize family involvement and reflect the diversity and complexity of interventions individualized for families. Drawing on a model of family-centered medical care in which Doherty and Baird (1987) defined services in terms of levels of practitioner involvement, Simeonsson and Bailey (1989) have proposed a comparable framework for conceptualizing levels of involvement for families in early intervention, displayed in Table 1. The hierarchical approach is designed to reflect qualitatively different levels of the nature and intensity of services sought by, and provided for, the family. The lowest level reflects the availability of services which the family elects not to access, while the highest level encompasses comprehensive therapeutic services addressing dynamic needs of the family. The ordinal conceptualization of the levels of involvement implies that higher levels potentially incorporate all services and provisions of lower levels. Thus, a family that is involved in dealing with strengthening a support network may also seek information and secure therapy for their child.

The above hierarchical model of levels of early intervention services and corresponding levels of family involvement leads to several considerations in design and conductance of evaluation studies. The first pertains to specificity of the evaluation question, and thus the nature of the dependent variables assessed, in terms of the nature and level of family involvement. For example, if the focus of services has been on meeting a family's needs for information, the evaluation question might address the extent to which parents were satisfied with the information received or whether it helped them make decisions on to achieve other outcomes or services. On the other hand, if the focus of services was on dealing with value conflicts within the family, evaluation would likely assess the extent to which problem-solving strategies were used or communication was improved. A second implication of this hierarchical model is that since intervention is seen as mutually determined by family and interventionist, evaluation of interven-

Table 11.1: Hierarchical dimensions of family involvement in
early intervention

LEVEL	DIMENSIONS OF INVOLVEMENT	EXAMPLE
0	Elective non-involvement	Family elects not to be involved in available services
I	Passive involvement	Family agrees to be identified and tracked
II	Neutral involvement	Family accesses developmental stimulation and allied therapies for child
III	Active formal involvement focusing on information needs	Family acquires information and skills to work with child
IV	Active personal involvement to secure/ extend personal and social support	Family secures and strengthens informal/ formal support network
V	Active behavioural involvement to define and deal with reality burdens	Family participates in partnership to identify, prioritize and implement interventions
VI	Active psychological involvement to define and deal with value conflicts	Family accesses comprehensive therapeutic services

tion should encompass both perspectives. Since parents and professionals are likely to enter the service arena with different goals for treatment and different values (Bailey, 1987), evaluation questions will need to assess the extent to which each party perceives the intervention to be successful. A final implication is a recognition of the intensity of involvement as a variable that should be accounted for in evaluation. The intensity of involvement limits the effects that can be expected and may be an important factor influencing the intensity of assessment measures and strategies.

In summary, a hierarchical model contributes to greater clarity and precision in evaluation. Essentially, the model argues that 'early intervention' is not a single, defined treatment that is applied equally to all children and families. Rather it is diverse in both scope and intensity, depending upon individualized family desires, the documented needs of children, and the availability of appropriate services. Given the extraordinary variability likely to be found in services, it is likely that the term 'early intervention' will be defined questionably as the unique set of services provided for each individual child and family. To expect that a single set of evaluation questions or outcome measures could adequately summarize this diversity may be unrealistic.

LEVELS OF CERTAINTY

One approach to achieving greater clarity and precision in the approach to evaluation might be complemented by improved clarity in the levels of evidence. By and large, evaluation studies in early intervention have focused on certainty of an effect or outcome in terms of statistical evidence. This, of course, is not always readily accomplished, which may account for the frequency of equivocal findings in the evaluation of early intervention programmes (Ottenbacher, 1989). The very nature of the phenomena under investigation in early intervention may dictate that other levels of evidence be considered. Addressing a comparable problem in the area of health evaluation, Smith (1981) proposes that evaluation may well involve evidence that is less than conclusive. Smith further argues that evaluation involving less than conclusive evidence may not only be sufficient but may, in some cases, be the only realistic alternative in such contexts.

While the effort to document real or perceived intervention impact in early intervention has typically sought conclusive evidence, evaluation of such impact, in future studies, might be improved by adopting a frameworking recognizing variable levels of certainty of evidence. This premise builds on the recognition that increased family involvement and increasingly complex interventions require an evaluation approach that takes into account corresponding levels of evidence. It may be useful in this context to explore frameworks which can substitute for, or complement, those based on scientific criteria with emphasis on statistical certainty. As noted above in the evaluation of human services, where the purpose often is practical management and decision making, the framework of law may constitute an attractive alternative (Smith, 1981). Drawing on the issues involved in health evaluation, Smith proposes that a consideration of levels of certainty allows an approach in evaluation in which evidence at lesser levels of certainty is 'sometimes acceptable and certainly better than no informed conclusions at all' (p. 278). To this end, Smith has drawn on the framework of law and identified three levels of evidence with relevance in health evaluations. These levels of certainty are defined in terms of suggestive, preponderant and conclusive evidence.

Level I certainty is defined as suggestive evidence, in which the degree of proof '...merely establishes that certain events, processes, or outcomes are plausible and within the realm of possible experience' (p. 274). As Smith indicates, suggestive evidence is the weakest form of evidence but may often be all that is available in formative phases. Level I certainty, however, only establishes the possibility of a relationship between treatment and outcome, and should be replaced by evidence of a greater level of certainty. Level II certainty, or preponderant evidence, is defined in terms of evaluation proof that '...not only is an event, process or outcomes possible, but that it more likely occurred than not' (p. 274). Preponderant evidence draws on cumulative information to support the conclusion that a relationship between treatment and outcomes is probably true. Conclusive evidence defines the final level of certainty — Level III, in which events or outcomes are undoubtedly true. Conclusive evidence is what is sought in well controlled experiments. In the field of law it is, according to Smith (1981), the level of evidence which leads to a conclusion which is beyond a shadow of doubt. It is interesting to note that the levels of certainty of evidence are conceptually very similar to levels of certainty of knowledge with norms, maxims, and principles paralleling suggestive, preponderant and conclusive evidence respectively (Bailey, 1988).

There are at least three important implications to a level of certainty framework, applied when evaluating early intervention programme impact. First, viewing evidence within a level of certainty framework makes it possible to expand programme evaluation beyond traditional experimental designs. Second, differentiating suggestive, preponderant, and conclusive evidence lends itself to events and outcomes in early intervention which vary in precision and certainty. A third implication is that a level of certainty framework provides an approach whereby the qualifications of evaluation findings can be formalized.

In implementing a level of certainty framework in evaluation of early intervention impact, the first step is to document the certainty of measurement. Once the certainty of measurement is determined, the degree to which interventions were implemented must be assessed. As Dobson and Cook (1980) have indicated, it is commonly assumed in evaluation studies that prescribed interventions and services are actually delivered. This assumption is open to question. Illustrating the problem of variability of implementation in human services, Dobson and Cook reported results from a field experiment which demonstrated that there was a functional relationship between programme outcomes and degree of implementation of services. The authors emphasized that 'if treatments are not delivered in a way which is consistent with programme objectives, it is likely evaluation efforts will be less than useful or, perhaps, meaningless' (Dobson and Cook, 1980, p. 270). An unfortunate outcome of this relationship for early intervention impact is that intervention may be judged as ineffective when the issue is in fact one of ineffective implementation.

LEVELS OF CERTAINTY IN EARLY INTERVENTION

The issue of levels of certainty is thus one with implications not only for evaluation evidence but also for the related aspects of precision of measurement and degree of implementation of interventions. A comprehensive approach for considering levels of certainty across these domains of early intervention is presented in Table II. For each domain, a specific level of certainty can be defined in terms of quality and precision. As Smith (1981) has indicated, there is a direct relationship between level of certainty or degree of proof and the quality of the evidence. In a more general sense, level of certainty can be increased if 'alternative conclusions have been eliminated; systematic bias or error have been eliminated; contextual factors have been approximately accounted for; assumptions made were accurate; most relevant variables and relationships were examined; all salient audience perspectives were considered; evidence was first-hand and material rather than circumstantial or hearsay' (Smith, 1981, p. 274).

Approaching evaluation of programme impact on the basis of the above framework implies that the level of certainty in evaluation is qualified by the nature and degree of implementation of intervention and the levels of certainty of measurement. Drawing on the descriptions in Table 2, it may be useful to illustrate distinctions in levels of certainty for one of the forms of intervention for families with handicapped infants. Within the hierarchical formats described in Table 2, a common intervention might be the family's active involvement in acquiring teaching and mangement skills (Level 3) with their handicapped child. Having defined the nature of intervention, it may be informative to examine the measurement, implementation and evaluation evidence associated with successive levels of certainty in the design and evaluation of this intervention as illustrated in Table 3. A review of the table indicates that increases in the level of certainty can be achieved with increased objectivity and validity of measurement, increased documentation of implementation and increased technical evidence in evaluation. This incremental approach is consistent with Offord's (1982) description of quality of evidence in evaluation, ranging from the lowest grade involving descriptive studies and opinions based on clinical experience to randomized trials. An

Table 11.2: Levels of certainty in early intervention domains

LEVELS OF CERTAINTY	DEFINITION	ASSESSMENT / MEASUREMENT DOMAIN	IMPLEMENTATION DOMAIN	EVALUATION DOMAIN
Suggestive evidence	Phenomena are plausible, possible	Subjective assessment	Documentation based on informal judgement	Several explanations for are possible
Preponderant evidence	Phenomena are probable	Objective assessment	Document base on available evidence	Competing explanations for change are reduced
Conclusive evidence	Phenomena are undoubetedly true	Multi/method, multi/perspective assessment: reliability and validity established	Documentation based on formal evidence collected systematically	Competing explanation for change are ruled out

examination of the impact of an intervention programme within this framework allows a consideration of what is desirable and what is feasible. As Smith (1981) has pointed out, the lower the level of certainty the more likely it is that an erroneous conclusion will be reached.

Specifying the level of certainty desired for a given programme would vary as a function of the purpose for evaluation and the resources available for designing and evaluating the programme. In some instances it may well be that suggestive evidence is acceptable for some decisions, whereas in others preponderant or conclusive evidence is seen as essential. Furthermore, it is also likely that different levels of evidence may be accepted for different domains within the evaluation of a programme. For example, the lack of attrition in family involvement may be seen as suggestive evidence of family satisfaction with services whereas independent observation of enhanced parent-child interaction may be seen as conclusive evidence.

Determination of the level of certainty appropriate in the evaluation of a given programme needs to take into account the design and the potential effects of the intervention. As a general rule, Smith (1981) has proposed that greater levels of certainty are indicated in a programme (a) when clients are at increased risk; (b) with increased intervention expense and (c) when the nature of the intervention is not readily understood or controlled. He has listed ten factors which can be used in determining the level of certainty suitable for a given intervention. Five of these pertain to the design of the programme with a greater need for certainty indicated, for example, if the programme is expensive, if participants are children or non-competent adults and if they are at some increased risk. The other five pertain to possible effects with a greater need for certainty indicated, for example, if the programme is expensive, if participants are children or non-competent adults and if they are at some increased risk. The other five pertain to possible effects with a greater need for certainty indicated for example if the number of beneficiaries is high, side effects are unknown and intervention effects are major. A review of these would be helpful in developing a comprehensive plan to design and evaluate interventions.

Table 11.3: Levels of certainty: Illustrating an application in Level III family involvement

LEVELS OF CERTAINTY	ASSESSMENT / MEASUREMENT DOMAIN	IMPLEMENTATION DOMAIN	EVALUATION DOMAIN
Suggestive evidence	Family's informational needs inferred from informal contacts	Information and training for family provided without monitoring	Informal family reports of satisfaction and acquisition of skills
Preponderant evidence	Family's informational needs explored in structured interview	Information and training for family provided according to planned format	Family's perception and reports of change documented formally
Conclusive evidence	Family's informational needs documented objectively from several members	Provision of information and training implementation with objective documentation	Objective measurement of change obtained; ruling out alternative explanations

CONCLUSIONS

In conclusion, the incremental growth of early intervention initiatives and the broadening scope of infant and family interventions are testimony to the intrinsic appeal and widely held belief that such intervention is effective. Attempts to apply traditional experimental designs and statistical procedures to document such effectiveness has yielded less than conclusive evidence, continuing the debate about the impact and efficiency of the preventive and interventive benefits of this approach. This chapter has proposed that this debate can be approached in two ways. Looking at early intervention as a field, it may be important to ask whether an exclusive search for conclusive evidence is either productive or warranted given the nature of the phenomena. In the context of the levels described by Smith (1981), it is reasonable to infer that effectiveness of programmes may in fact more appropriately be documented by suggestive or preponderant evidence. A second way in which the debate may be approached is to explore the utility of alternate conceptualizations of evidence beyond the prevailing statistical approach. In so doing, it may be possible to bring about a rapprochement between demands for accountability and a realistic appraisal of the complexity of evaluating impact of human services.

SUMMARY OF MAIN POINTS

1. Evaluating the impact of early intervention has yieled equivocal evidence because studies have often been inadequate with respect to experimental rigour, sample size and outcome measures.
2. It can be argued that the premise for providing early intervention should rest on clinical and humanitarian grounds rather than empirical grounds.
3. Early intervention embraces a diverse and complex range of services, particularly when consideration is given to the nature and intensity of services sought by, and provided for, the family. A hierarchical model which portrays varying dimensions of family involvement serves to illustrate this diversity.

4. The framework of law provides a different, and perhaps more appropriate, model for evaluating early intervention programmes. In this model, three levels of evidence are considered: suggestive, preponderant and conclusive evidence. Such an approach takes account of the fact that events and outcomes in early intervention are inherently varied in precision and certainty. In some instances suggestive evidence would be acceptable, whereas in other preponderant or conclusive evidence would be essential.

REFERENCES

Bailey, D.B. and Simeonsson, R.J. (1986) 'Design issues in family impact evaluation,' in L. Bickman and D.L. Weatherford (eds), *Evaluating Early Intervention Programmes for Severely Handicapped Children and Their Families*, Pro-Ed, Austin, TX.

Casto, G. and Mastropieri, M.A. (1986) 'The efficacy of early intervention programs: A meto-analysis,' *Exceptional Children*, 52, 417–424.

Dobson, D. and Cook, T.J. (1980) 'Avoiding type III error in program evaluation,' *Evaluation and Program Planning*, 3, 269–276.

Doherty, W.T. and Baird, M.A. (1987) *Family Centered Medical Care: A Clinical Casebook*, Guilford Press, New York.

Dunst, C. (1985) 'Editors introduction', *Analysis and Intervention in Developmental Disabilities*, 5, 1–5.

Dunst, C. and Snyder, S. (1987) 'A critique of the Utah State University early intervention meta-analysis research,' *Exceptional Children*, 53(3), 260–265.

Hanson, M.J. (1985) 'An analysis of the effects of early intervention services for infants and toddlers with moderate and severe handicaps,' *Topics in Early Childhood Special Education*, 5, 36–51.

Meisels, S.J. (1985) 'The efficacy of early intervention: Why are we still asking this question?' *Topics in Early Childhood Education*, 5(2), 1–11.

Offord, G.R. (1982) 'Primary prevention: Aspects of program design and evaluation,' *Journal of the American Academy of Child Psychiatry*, 21(1), 225–230.

Ottenbacher, K.J. (1989) 'Statistical conclusion validity of early intervention research with handicapped children,' *Exceptional Children*, 55(6), 534–540.

Shonkoff, J.P. and Hauser-Cram, P. (1987) 'Early intervention for disabled infants and their families: A quantitative analysis,' *Pediatrics*, *80*(5), 650–658.

Simeonsson, R.J. and Bailey, D.B. (1989), 'Family dimensions in early intervention,' in S.J. Meisels and J.P. Shonkoff (eds), *Handbook of Early Childhood Intervention*, Cambridge University Press, Boston.

Smith, N.L. (1981) 'The certainty of judgments in health evaluations,' *Evaluation and Program Planning*, *4*, 273–278.

Strain, P. and Smith, B.J. (1987) A counter-interpretation of early intervention effects a response to Casto and Mastropieri,' *Exceptional Children*, *53*(3), 260–265.

Vadasy, P.F., Fewell, R.R., Greenberg, M.T., Dermond, N.L., and Meyer, D.J. (1986) 'Follow-up evaluation of the effect of involvement in the father's program,' *Topics in Early Childhood Special Education*, *6*, 16–31.

12 DESIGNING AND EVALUATING EARLY INTERVENTION PROGRAMMES

David R. Mitchell

INTRODUCTION

Early intervention for infants and toddlers with handicaps and their families is increasingly recognized as an essential component of a modern society's special education services. During the past decade there has been a trend in many countries to provide a comprehensive range of provisions for this population — a trend that represents the confluence of several factors: a recognition of the importance of early experiences for the development of handicapped and at-risk children, the emergence of technologies for working with such children, parental advocacy, and accumulating evidence as to the efficacy of early intervention (Mitchell, Brynelsen and Holm, 1988).

This expansion of early intervention services has not necessarily reflected an explicit agreement as to which of the many competing models of service delivery should prevail. Thus, programmes are diverse with respect to their policies and practices in a range of areas, including the agencies which control them, the nature of their clientele, their modes of service delivery, curricula, assessment methods, relationship with parents, and so on. In the past few years, however, this diversity has begun to give way to a common philosophy as to what constitutes optimal early intervention. This emerging consensus reflects several factors: a shared value system as to the rights of disabled and at-risk children, the impact of an international literature of research findings and programme ideas, and the growing network of contacts among parents and professionals working in this field (Mitchell, Brynelsen and Holm, 1988).

One of the major issues in the development of early intervention services has been the question of how best to evaluate their quality (Guralnick and Bennett, 1987; Simeonsson and Bailey in this volume discuss this in some detail). Much of the evaluation work to date has been focused on the outcome of early intervention programmes, but very little attention has been paid to evaluating processes. Further, the emphasis has been on summative, rather than formative, evaluation.

The thrust of this chapter will be on the importance of developing a comprehensive evaluation strategy which attends to process as well as outcome evaluation and formative as well as summative evaluation. The central thesis is that programme evaluation and programme design are the reciprocals of each other. In other words, evaluation should lead to improved programme design. Or, as Shadish (1986) has pointed out, 'evaluation... can be no better than the change process in which it is embedded'.

The remainder of this chapter is divided into three major sections. Firstly, there will be an overview of principles underlying programme evaluation, with an emphasis on developing a model to show the relationships between programme inputs, goals, design and evaluation. Secondly, there will be a description of the rationale, structure and administration of a scale for evaluating early intervention programmes. A final section will present conclusions and a summary of the principal points.

PRINCIPLES OF PROGRAMME EVALUATION

This chapter advocates an approach to evaluating early intervention programmes that brings together two principal thrusts. Firstly, it is argued that evaluation of programmes should reflect an understanding of its relationships to programme inputs, goals and design. This notion of a linked system, advocated in general terms by Bagnato and Neisworth (1981), has been applied to the field of early intervention by Bricker and her colleagues who have advocated 'a strong and continuing linkage from assessment to IEP development to curricular emphasis to evaluation' (Bricker, 1986; Notari, Slentz and Bricker, this volume).

The second thesis is that evaluation of a programme should not only focus on fact questions, but should not only focus on fact questions, but should also be concerned with value questions (Dokecki, 1986; Smith, 1986). This expansion of the notion of programme evaluation into the domain of values has led to a recent interest in evaluating the quality of early intervention programmes' operations relative to criteria of best practices (Mitchell, Brynelsen, and Holm, 1988).

These themes come together in the model of evaluation portrayed in Figure 1. This model shows the two threads of evaluation — outcome and process — and the relationships among programme inputs, goals, design and evaluation. The elements of this model will be discussed in the remainder of this section.

Needs Assessment

Since the prime purpose of an early intervention programme is to meet the needs of its clients, it is necessary to obtain comprehensive baseline data on these needs upon a family's entry into the programme. For children, such assessments typically involve ascertaining their level of functioning in such areas as cognition, language, motor skills, social skills and self care (Bricker, 1986; US Department of Education, 1987). Systematic assessment of family functioning has emerged only recently (Bailey and Simeonsson, 1986; Fewell, 1986; Kysela *et al.*, 1987; Seligman, 1983) and tends to focus on such factors as needs, stress, social supports, levels of sat-

Figure 12.1: Evaluation model.

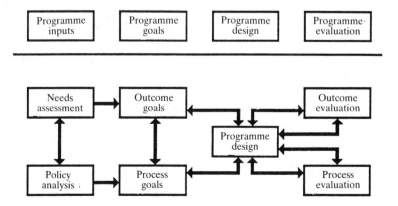

isfaction with services, parent's roles, and family interaction patterns. As well as a recognition of the importance of comprehensiveness, two other features of needs assessment stand out. Firstly, because they usually form the basis of intervention programmes, criterion-referenced, rather than norm-referenced, tests are preferred (Ballard, this volume; Bricker, 1986). Criterion-referenced tests allow one to more accurately ascertain a child's progress in achieving certain targeted functional skills against his or her baseline performances on those skills (Peterson, 1987). Secondly, because the range of skills concerned in comprehensive needs assessments are usually beyond the competence of any single professional, there is a growing consensus that such assessments should be carried out by multidisciplinary teams (Bricker, 1986; US Department of Education, 1987).

Policy analysis

As well as input resulting from the needs assessment of its clients, a programme is subjected to other influences. Some of these are quite explicit, others are more subtle. Some originate in the broader society in which the programme operates, others are present in the theories and values of the professionals and administrators associated with the programme.

Four principal sources of policy inputs may be identified:

1. *Legal requirements* — Clearly, a programme must be aware of and responsive to the laws of the society in which it operates. In the United States, for example, the recent introduction of PL 99-457 will have a profound effect on early intervention programmes in that country. This 1986 amendment to the Education of All Handicapped Children Act aims at assisting states to establish statewide systems of early intervention services for infants and toddlers with handicaps and their families. Among its many features, this act defines eligibility for early intervention, requires the setting up of public awareness programmes and comprehensive child find systems, and lays down requirements for individualized family service plans.

2. *Consumer demands* — Organizations representing disabled persons and their families continue to have a major input into special educational services. Because parents are typically closely involved in early intervention programmes, attending to their input is a particular responsibility of programme designers.

3. *Research findings* — During the past decade there has been a dramatic expansion of the literature on early intervention, with publications covering such areas as research into its effectiveness (e.g., Guralnick and Bennett, 1987), programme design (Bricker, 1986; Peterson, 1987), evaluation (Bickman and Weatherford, 1986), and families (Fewell, 1986; Seligman, 1983). Although there is considerable diversity of views as to what constitutes the specific features of best practices, even across diverse cultures a consensus seems to be evolving with respect to broad principles (Mitchell, Brynelsen and Holm, 1988; Subregional Workshop for Commonwealth Countries of South-East-Central Africa, 1987). It is therefore timely that these threads be drawn together to suggest broad guidelines for designing and evaluating early intervention programmes.

4. *Staff members' philosophies* — Professionals and administrators bring to a programme their personal sets of social values and theories regarding intervention. Sometimes these philosophies are quite explicit, sometimes they are implicit in the actions individually or collectively undertaken (or not undertaken) by the staff. As far as early intervention is concerned, some of the most dramatic differences can be found in the distinction between a child vs. the whole family orientation, behavioural vs. developmental theories, curricula which anticipate a child's developmental needs vs. those which are responsive to a child's interests and environment, and a separatist vs. integrationist approach to working with disabled and at-risk children. Again, it behoves programme designers and evaluators to take these factors into account.

Programme Goals

Early intervention programmes usually focus their activities around outcome goals they hold for individual children and their families. Only occasionally do they specify goals associated with the processes of the programme. These two types of goals — which, it must be emphasized, interact with each other — will be discussed below.

Outcome goals — The needs assessment phase of programme development, as noted earlier, should yield data on the needs and strengths of individual children and their families. During this goal-setting phase, individual education plans (IEPs) and/or individualized family service plans (IFSPs) should be prepared. These plans should contain both long-term goals and more immediate objectives, as well as a specification of the criteria, procedures and timelines that will be used to determine progress toward achieving outcome goals (US Department of Education, 1987).

Process goals — In addition to determining outcome goals for its clients, a programme should also determine what processes it will employ to achieve these outcomes. As noted earlier, process goals reflect the values, beliefs and theories that characterize a programme — sometimes explicitly stated, but more often implicit in the activities of a programme. One of the most systematic attempts derived from this source. These six process goals are as follows:

1. *Community coherence* — The programme enhances the social coherence and solidarity of community by recognizing and asserting that persons with disabilities have the right to be full and effective participants in the community.

2. *Cultural sensitivity* — The programme is sensitive to and supportive of cultural pluralism and ensures that its goals and processes are culturally and ecologically valid.

3. *Right to services* — The programme recognizes and asserts that persons with disabilities have the right to services that will help them develop to their potential.

4. *Family integrity* — The programme strengthens the family by

respecting its integrity, by enhancing the competence of its members, by helping its members to access resources appro priate to the needs of persons with disabilities, and by recog nizing its uniqueness.

5. *Professional standards* — The programme seeks to achieve the highest professional standards in the design and implemen tation of its work.

6. *Accountability* — The programme is accountable for the effi cient management of its resources.

Programme Design

In order to achieve its outcome and process goals, a programme must establish procedures and structures. Typically, these involve making decisions on questions in the following broad areas:

Social policies — What position should the programme take with respect to such values as community coherence, cultural sensitivity, rights, and family integrity, as discussed in the previ ous section? How should these positions be reflected in other aspects of the programme design? How should the policies be promulgated within the programme and the broader community?

Administration and management — What principles of man agement should be followed? To whom should administration of the programme be ultimately responsible? Who should fund the programme? What role should parents play in the management of the programme? How should staff be trained and how should their professional development be continued? What form of record-keeping should be employed? How can services be coor dinated in particular communities in order to avoid undesirable duplication and to plan for future developments?

Physical environment — Should the programme include a centre-based component, and if so, where should it be located and how should it be designed?

Curricula — What broad philosophical position(s) regarding the structure of curricula should be adopted? What should be the scope of any curricula? Should curricula be developed for families as well as for individual children? What is the appropriate balance between anticipatory and responsive curricula? Structured and unstructured curricula?

Teaching/therapy strategies and methods — What theoretical approaches to learning and teaching should be adopted? Should parents play a role in developing and implementing teaching/therapy programmes for their children and, if so, how should this role be defined? What are the most effective professional-parent relationships?

Programme Evaluation

Programme evaluation takes place when there is a systematic attempt to ascertain the extent to which a programme has achieved its goals and objectives. Before embarking on an evaluation, three broad strategy decisions have to be made. Firstly, is the focus to be on a programme's outcomes or its processes? Secondly, is the evaluation intended to serve summative or formative goals? Thirdly, who should be responsible for the evaluation: the programme staff alone, external consultants alone, or some combination of the two?

Outcome and Process Evaluation

The prime purpose of outcome evaluation is to determine the extent to which the goals and objectives held for individual children and their families are being met. Related to this is a concern for ascertaining whether the programme, as a whole, is functioning successfully (see Guralnick and Bennett, 1987, for a comprehensive review of research in this area).

The purpose of process evaluation is to determine the extent to which all aspects of the early intervention model (including outcome evaluation procedures) are in place. This involves evaluating the extent to which a programme's policies and practices conform to criteria subsumed under various aspects of the model portrayed in Figure 1. Data on these issues are usually obtained through observations of the programme in action, interviews of professional and administrative staff and parents, and inspection of the programme's documentation.

Summative and Formative Evaluation

Sometimes programme evaluation has the purpose of making judgments about the appropriateness of a child or family continuing with a programme or about the value of a programme. This focus on accountability characterizes what is referred to as summative evaluation. In contrast, formative evaluation is concerned with measuring performances (in the case of outcome evaluation) and/or policies and practices (in the case of process evaluation) with a view to deciding on modifications to programme design. In Figure 1, the formative approach to evaluation is portrayed in the feedback loops which extend from programme evaluation to programme design.

Internal, External and Conjoint Evaluation

Evaluation can further be characterized in terms of who carries it out: the programme staff alone (internal), outside consultants alone (external), or programme staff in collaboration withoutside consultants (conjoint). (See Hughson and Brown, 1988; Mitchell, Brynelsen and Holm, 1988; for further comments on conjoint evaluation.)

The following section of the chapter describes a scale which has been developed to guide the conjoint and formative evaluation of the process aspects of early intervention programmes.

A SCALE FOR EVALUATING EARLY INTERVENTION PROGRAMMES

This section of the chapter will present a detailed discussion of a 51-item scale which can be used as a basis for designing and evaluating early intervention programmes. The scale conforms with the two principles underlying the model shown in Figure 1, namely that attention should be paid to both process and outcome variables and that there should be strong linkages among programme inputs, goals, design, and evaluation.

The discussion is organized under the following headings:

1. development of the scale,
2. rationale of the scale,
3. structure of the scale,
4. administration of the scale,
5. scoring the scale,
6. application of the scale.

Development of the Scale

The development of the scale spanned a two-year period from 1986 to 1988. The first draft had its origins in the writer's experience in directing a university-based early intervention programme for young children with Down's Syndrome and their families, his participation in setting up a community-based programme, his observations of programmes in Australia, Canada, New Zealand, United Kingdom, and USA, and extensive searches of the literature on early intervention. This process yielded a series of criteria which, in the writer's opinion, constituted 'best practices' of early intervention programmes.

These criteria were then circulated to a sample of New Zealand and Canadian professionals working in early intervention. Their feedback, together with the experiences gained from preliminary field trials in Canada and New Zealand, led to the development of a further draft. This was then circulated to an international sample of people who were prominently involved in early intervention in Australia (6), Canada (5), New Zealand (17), UK/Ireland (5), and USA (6). These 39 respondents came from a variety of backgrounds: 21 were drawn from tertiary education/ research, 15 were directly involved in early intervention programmes and four were parents or parent groups. This survey took the form of asking respondents to rate a total of 51 items on a four-point scale, according to the following criteria:

1. An essential component which should be given a high weighting
2. An essential component which should be given a moderate weighting
3. A desirable, but not essential, component which should be given a low weighting
4. Not appropriate for inclusion in a scale.

Median rankings were then calculated for each of the items, this information leading to a decision to delete two items. Comments from the respondents led to two new items being added and slight amendments being made to the wording of some items to clarify their intent.

During 1987, extensive field trials were carried out with the draft that emerged from the process described above. These were conducted in three main locations (New Zealand: eight programmes; British Columbia: eight programmes; The Gaza Strip: one programme with 30 staff members). As a result of these trials, the scoring categories were clarified, further minor changes were made to the wording of some criteria and two items were merged. The version of the scale that emerged from this process comprised 50 items. In 1988, final revisions to the scale were carried out in the United States where the writer consulted with early intervention workers and took PL 99-457 regulations (US Department of Education, 1987) into account. A new item was added as a result of this process. As well, the scale was reconciled with a series of recommendations from a group of developing countries (Sub-regional Workshop for Commonwealth Countries of South-East-Central Africa, 1987).

Rationale of the Scale

As outlined earlier, the writer advocates an approach to evaluation which gives consideration to process as well as outcomes and to the linkages among programme inputs, goals, design, and evaluation. In addition, the following six value positions underpin the scale: community coherence, cultural sensitivity, right to services, family integrity, professional standards, and accountability. While it is possible to use the scale either for summative or formative evaluation purposes, the writer strongly advocates the latter use.

Structure of the Scale

The scale comprises a total of 51 criteria against which the policies and practices of early intervention programmes for young children with special needs (YCWSN) are evaluated. These criteria are arranged under 14 broad headings and cover such areas as the curricula, assessment, staff training, parent–professional relationship, and administration. In order to illustrate the character of the scale, items from each of the 14 major areas, together with brief descriptions of the underlying values and examples of references relevant to the content of the items, are presented below.

A. Children Served by the Programme (three items)

Example:
> The programme serves children with a broad range of disabilities and significant at-risk features and is not restricted to children classified as belonging to a narrow range of traditional, medically-oriented disability categories. Thus, the programme will describe itself as being concerned with 'developmentally delayed children' or 'children with learning difficulties' or 'children with special needs'.

Underlying Value: #1 Community coherence.

References: Mitchell (1983), US Department of Education (1987), Vincent *et al.* (1986), Warnock (1978).

B. <u>Assessment</u> (four items)

Example

Children's performances on a broad range of skill areas are regularly assessed by programme staff (at least every six months).

Underlying Value: #5 Professional standards.

References: Accreditation Council for Services for Mentally Retarded and other Developmentally Disabled Persons (1984), Bricker (1986), Brynelsen (1984), Guralnick and Bricker (1987), Hupp and Kaiser (1986), Pieterse (1985), US Department of Education (1987), Warnock (1978).

C. <u>The Curricula</u> (seven items)

Example

The programme includes strategies for enhancing the quality of parent–child interactions, both in terms of (a) social relationships and (b) communication, and it uses materials and curricula designed to improve the quality of parent–child interactions. To this end, it includes a concern for encouraging parents to be responsive to children's initiations.

Underlying values: #4 Family integrity and #5 Professional standards.

References: Barrera and Rosenbaum (1986), Bromwich (1981), Guralnick and Bennett (1987), Honig (1982), Kysela *et al.* (1987), Manolson (1983), Marfo and Kysela (1985), Mitchell (1987), Rosenberg and Robinson (1985).

D. Counselling and Support (four items)

Example
> The programme takes account of the needs that some
> families, individual parents and other family members
> have for individual or group counselling. Where appropri-
> ate, and where the family member(s) concerned wish it,
> counselling is given by professionals working in the pro-
> gramme or they assist parents to receive counselling from
> professionals working in other agencies.

Underlying value: #4 Family integrity.
References: Bricker (1986), Gabel, McDowell and Cerreto (1983),
Kysela *et al.* (1987), Seligman (1983).

E. Advocacy (two items)

Example
> The programme staff and its management committee seek
> out and/or respond to opportunities to act as advocates for
> the rights of YCWSN and their families, especially on
> issues that are within their professional expertise and
> where such advocacy does not preempt the role of parents.

Underlying value: #3 Right to services.

References: Filler (1983).

F. Transdisciplinary Approaches (two items)

Example
> Where the programme is staffed by several professionals,
> one team member is assigned primary liaison responsibili-
> ties for each YCWSN and his or her family.

Underlying value: #4 Family integrity.

References: Accreditation Council for Services for Mentally Retarded and other Developmentally Disabled Persons (1984), Bricker
(1986), Fewell (1983), Orelove and Sobsey (1987), US Department
of Education (1987).

G. Staff Training (four items)

Example

    The professionals employed in the programme have received pre-employment (pre-service) training which includes relevant specialized post-secondary (tertiary level) preparation for working with YCWSN and their families.

Underlying value: #5 Professional standards.

References: Brynelsen (1984), Guralnick and Bennett (1987), Pieterse (1985), US Department of Education (1987), Warnock (1978).

H. Programme Evaluation (three items)

Example

    The programme regularly and objectively evaluates the impact of its work with its clients. Such evaluation uses instruments which reflect the range of goals held for individual YCWSN and their families and the specific processes employed in the programme. This evaluation is directed at discovering the overall strengths and weaknesses of the programme.

Underlying value: #6 Accountability.

References: Bickman and Weatherford (1986), Bricker (1986), Dunst (1985), Filler (1983), Guralnick and Bennett (1987), Marfo and Kysela (1985), Straton (1985), Wolery and Bailey (1984).

I. Cultural Sensitivity (two items)

Example
> The programme is sensitive and responsive to cultural
> differences among families in the community it serves.
> This is reflected, for example, in the consideration given to
> (a) the language backgrounds of YCWSN and their fami-
> lies, (b) the values of different cultural groups, (c) the per-
> ceptions of handicap or disability held by different cultural
> groups, and (d) cultural differences in parent–child interac-
> tions.

Underlying value: #2 Cultural sensitivity.

References: Accreditation Council for Services for Mentally Retarded and other Developmentally Disabled Persons (1984), Hosaka (1984), Mayfield (1986), US Department of Education (1987),
Westby (1988).

J. Interagency Coordination (two items)

Example
> There is an effective transition procedure of YCWSN as
> they move from the programme to an appropriate pre-
> school facility, or to school. These procedures include
> (a) exploring placement options with parents, (b) transmit-
> ting appropriate records on individual children and details
> of the programme's philosophies and procedures, (c) en-
> suring that the parents of the YCWSN have opportunities
> to observe the facilities and to discuss them with the staff,
> and (d) supporting parents in making their placement
> decisions.

Underlying value: #4 Family integrity.

References: Bricker (1986), Brynelsen (1984), US Department of
Education (1987).

K. <u>Parent-professional Relationships</u> (three items)

Example

Parents and professionals in the programme work together in a partnership relationship in designing and implementing programmes for individual children. This relationship is characterized by (a) active and ongoing dialogue between parents and professionals, (b) professionals treating parents' contributions as important, and (c) a recognition on the part of professionals that, within the constraints imposed by the law, parents have ultimate responsibility for decisions affecting themselves and their children.

Underlying value: #4 Family integrity.

References: Bricker (1986), Brynelsen (1984), Filler (1983), Guralnick and Bricker (1987), Hupp and Kaiser (1986), Lillie (1981), Mittler, Mittler, and McConachie (1986), Warnock (1978).

L. Integration (two items)

Example

The programme includes opportunities for YCWSN and their parents to have significant contact with non-disabled children and their parents. This means (a) that if the programme is centre-based, a broad range of children, including YCWSN and their parents and non-disabled children and their parents attend the same sessions (b) if it is home-based, the programme staff actively encourages contact between YCWSN and their parents and non-disabled children and their parents, or (c) that the programme organizes opportunities for YCWSN to be enrolled in integrated pre-school settings.

Underlying value: #1 Community coherence.

References: Bricker (1986).

M. <u>Location and Physical Environment of Centre</u> (four items)

Example
>   The physical environment of the centre (in the case of
>   centre-based programmes) is adapted to take account of
>   the range of disabilities manifested by YCWSN.

Underlying value: #3 Right to services.

References: Bricker (1986), Hupp and Kaiser (1986).

N. Administration (eight items)

Example
>   The organization(s) responsible for administering the
>   programme and overseeing its standards includes indi-
>   viduals with professional expertise relevant to the activities
>   undertaken in the programme on the programme's man-
>   agement committee (board of directors) and/or on a pro-
>   fessional sub-committee (advisory committee).

Underlying value: #6 Accountability.

Administration of the Scale

As mentioned earlier, the writer recommends that the scale be
employed in formative evaluation, i.e. evaluation which has programme improvement as its main goal. It is also recommended
that this evaluation take place in the context of a consultancy
relationship between programme staff and administrators ('consultees') and external evaluators ('consultants') — a procedure
which is now outlined.

Principles of consultancy. The consultancy relationship is guided by
six maxims (Kemmis and McTaggart, 1982; Mannino and Shore,
1985; Mitchell, Brynelsen, and Holm, 1988):

1. The primary goal of the consultancy is to bring about and monitor improvements in the consultees' practices and in their understanding of their practices in working with their clients.
2. The consultants' role is to assist the consultees to develop an appropriate strategy to achieve the consultancy goal. They do this by providing advice on methodology, a set of process evaluation criteria, data derived from the evaluation, and advice and support on ways in which criteria may be met. Typically, this process involves the following cycle of activities:

   a) identifying the need to carry out a process evaluation consultancy
   b) planning the consultancy
   c) acting to bring about the consultancy
   d) obtaining relevant data
   e) reflecting on the data and its significance for bringing about programme improvements
   f) planning to bring about programme improvements
   g) acting to bring about changes in the consultees' practices and in their understanding of their practices
   h) obtaining further data.

3. The process evaluation consultancy takes place in the programme's natural environment.
4. The relationship between the consultants and consultees is characterized by a spirit of collaboration, openness and trust, with the consultees actively involved in all phases.
5. The data obtained in the consultancy are the consultees' intellectual property and are to be treated as confidential by the consultants unless otherwise negotiated.
6. The consulting process is time-limited and operates on the basis for a clear working plan.

The consultancy process. In keeping with the above principles, a typical consultancy using the scale involves the following steps:

1. *In advance of the consultancy*: questions of staff, board members and parents are sent to the programme for distribution and the purpose and character of the consultancy are summarized.
2. *The consultancy visit, Day 1*: The consultants (a) are oriented to the programme, (b) undertake a home visit and/or observe the centre, (c) collectively interview staff and representatives of the governing board on questions relating to items in the scale, (d) collectively interview two sets of parents (one nominated by the programme, the other chosen at random), and (e) view records and other documentation. The consultants and the consultees then independently rate the programme on the criteria specified in the scale.
3. *The consultancy visit, Day 2*: The consultants and the consultees 'negotiate' ratings for each of the 51 items on the scale, the procedure being chaired by one of the consultees. In the course of this meeting, suggestions for improving the programme are discussed.
4. *Short-term follow-up*: The consultants prepare a report which records the decisions and recommendations made during the consultancy visit and assist the programme staff to set up specific action plans, time-lines and areas of responsibility for implementing recommendation.
5. *Long-term follow-up*: Six months after the initial consultancy, the above cycle is repeated, with an emphasis on considering the items where the programme did not fully meet the criteria on the initial consultancy.

Scoring the Scale

Each item is scored according to the degree to which the programme's policies and practices meet the criterion. A four-point rating scale is used, each item being rated in terms of whether it:

    A. Fully meets the criterion.
    B. Largely meets the criterion.
    C. Meets the criterion to a small extent.
    D. Does not meet any aspect of the criterion.

Intermediate ratings (D+, C+, B+) are given if a policy and/or practice is actively under review and is likely to change in the direction of the criterion in the near future.

A further feature of the scoring is the possibility of excluding items if it was decided that they were inappropriate to the particular circumstances of the programme 'on grounds that would stand scrutiny by an independent panel'. This procedure should be used very sparingly.

The following is an example of an item from the scale, with the criterion, questions asked of staff and parents, and the scoring method:

#3 The programme actively seeks to discover young children with special needs for whom it may be able to offer an appropriate service. It does this by such means as (a) keeping key agencies and professionals informed of what it can offer, and (b) publicizing the programme in the community, taking particular care to ensure that families who are disadvantaged economically who live in isolated areas or whose cultural or language backgrounds might prevent them from becoming aware of services have access to information on the programme.

Questions: Staff

3.1 How do you publicize your services in the community?
3.2 What steps do you take to ensure that key agencies/ professionals are informed?
3.3 What steps do you take to inform parents who are disadvantaged...?

Questions: Parents

3.4 How did you find out about the programme?

Scoring

A The programme fully meets all aspects of the criterion.

B   The programme effectively publicizes itself through agencies or professionals and in the broader community, but does little to ensure that minority groups have access to appropriate information on the programme.
C   The programme publicizes its services almost exclusively through agencies and professionals and takes few steps to publicize itself in the community.
D   The programme does very little to publicize its services, relying primarily on word of mouth.

Programme's Rating ( ) Evaluators' Rating ( ) Agreed Rating ( )

To illustrate the scoring of the scale, summaries of three programmes' performances on this item, together with the ratings that were agreed to, are presented below.

Programme #1. This programme publicized its services by means such as the following: talks are given to parent support groups, personal contacts are regularly (at least annually) made with key agencies working with families (e.g. community health nurses who see 98% of all babies in the area), brochures on the programme are distributed to agencies and paediatricians, information on the programme is regularly inserted in health bulletins which have a wide distribution among health professionals, immigrant support groups are contacted, and brochures written in Punjabian are available for families from that background. Rating: A. Comment: This programme fully meets all aspects of the criterion.

Programme #2. This programme uses several means to publicize its services: it participates in biennial community health fairs, it distributes pamphlets on the programme to public health nurses and doctors (but the frequency was not known), and it distributes posters to health units and Ministry of Human Resources offices. It has received some publicity through newspapers and radio talk-back shows, but this has not occurred in the past couple of years. The programme's area includes a native Indian population of approximately 500 people. This group is served by a health nurse and a social worker with whom the programme staff liaise. However, the programme's materials are not specifically adapted to the native Indian culture.

Rating: B. Comment: While this programme regularly and effectively publicizes its services among professional groups and the broader community, it was agreed that more attempts should be made to publicize the programme among minority groups in the community.

Programme #3. This programme relies primarily on word of mouth contacts and on parents seeing cars with the society's symbols displayed. Doctors come on visits to the centre, but it is more than two years since the last such visits took place. No written publication on the programme is available.

Rating: D. Comment: For the most part, this programme relies on word of mouth to make its services known. While this is generally an effective way of communicating in a tightly-knit community such as _____, it was agreed that more systematic efforts should be made to ensure that potential clients find out as early as possible about the programme and that pamphlets describing its work should be prepared and regularly distributed among key agencies.

Applications of the Scale

To date, the scale has been used to evaluate eight programmes in New Zealand, eight in British Columbia, and one (with 30 programme staff) in the Gaza Strip. In all of these evaluations, the resulting profiles were used as a basis for planning improvements to the respective programmes. In the case of the British Columbia programmes, the results led to the development of in-service courses for staff.

Table 1 shows the distribution of the ratings achieved by programmes in the three locations. On average, programmes in British Columbia fully met 56 per cent of the criteria, compared with 36 per cent in the New Zealand programmes and 26 per cent in the Gaza Strip.

Table 12.1: Distribution of ratings across programmes (percentages)

Ratings	BC (*N*=8)	NZ (*N*=20)	Gaza (*N*=1)
Criteria fully met	56	38	26
Criteria mainly met	33	25	30
Criteria met to small extent	9	23	25
Criteria not met	2	14	9

Table 12.2 presents data on the extent to which the staff of the programme and the external evaluators agreed on their initial ratings of the programmes in British Columbia and New Zealand. It can be seen that on average, there was complete agreement on 69 per cent of the criteria, with one grade difference on 28% of the criteria and two to three grade differences for the remaining 4%.

Table 12.2: Extent of agreement between programme staff and external evaluators (percentages)

Level of agreement	BC (*N*=8)	NZ (*N*=8)	Total
Complete agreement	72	65	69
1 grade difference	26	30	28
2/3 grades difference	2	5	5

Table 12.3 shows the direction of the differences in ratings given by programme staff and external evaluators. It can be seen that where programme staff and evaluators differed in their ratings, the former gave their programmes higher ratings than external evaluators in a ratio of 2:1. Even so, it should not be overlooked that in one-third of the ratings where there were differences, the programme staff underestimated their programme's standing. This suggests that the processes employed were by no means inimical to self-criticism.

Table 12.3: Direction of difference in ratings by programme
staff and external evaluators (percentages)

Direction of differences	BC (N=8)	NZ (N=8)	Total
No differences	65	72	69
Programme staff higher	24	15	20
Evaluators higher	11	12	12

From Table 4 it can be seen that differences between evaluators and programme staff were resolved in the direction of the
former in a ratio of 2:1. In some cases, these resolutions arose from
clarification of the criteria (which have since been incorporated in
the manual for the scale); in others, they reflected differences in
judgment where the external evaluators succeeded in persuading
the programme staff to accept their views.

Table 12.4: Direction of resolution of differences in ratings
by programme staff and external evaluators (percentages)

Direction of resolution	BC (N=8)	NZ (N=8)	Total
No differences	65	72	69
Towards programme's ratings	10	12	11
Towards evaluators' ratings	25	15	20
Compromise	1	1	1

SUMMARY AND CONCLUSION

This chapter is divided into two broad sections; one devoted to a
discussion of general principles of programme evaluation, and the
second to a description of the rationale, structure and application
of a scale for evaluating early intervention programmes.

Seven broad recommendations arise from the material reviewed in this chapter:

1. The evaluation of early intervention programmes should be sufficiently comprehensive as to cover all aspects of a programme's inputs, goals and design features.

2. Evaluation should be concerned with examining value questions, as well as factual questions.

3. The following six broad values are presented as a sound basis for designing programmes: community coherence, cultural sensitivity, right to services, family integrity, professional standards and accountability.

4. Evaluation should focus on examining the quality of the processes employed in programmes, as well as on their outcomes.

5. While there is a place for summative evaluation, formative evaluation, with its emphasis upon assisting programme goals, is the preferred approach.

6. Evaluation is best carried out as a conjoint acitivity involving the collaboration between external consultants and the programme staff, with the latter taking primary responsibility for the decisions.

7. An internationally-validated scale for evaluating the process of early intervention programmes is presented as having utility for forming the basis of evaluations in different settings.

REFERENCES

Accreditation Council for Services for Mentally Retarded and other Developmentally Disabled Infants (1984) *Standards for Services for Developmentally Disabled Individuals*, ACMRD, Washington, DC.

Bagnato, S. and Neisworth, J. (1981) *Linking Developmental Assessment and Curricula*, Aspen, Rockville, Maryland.

Bailey, D.B. and Simeonsson, R.J. (1986) 'Design Issues in Family Impact Evaluation,' in L. Bickman & D.L. Weatherford (eds), *Evaluating Early Intervention Programmes for Severely Handicapped Children and Their Families*, Pro-ed, Austin.

Barrera, M. E. and Rosenbaum, P. (1986) 'The Transactional Model of Early Home Intervention,' *Infant Mental Health Journal, 7*, 112–131.

Bickman, L. and Weatherford, D. L. (eds) (1986) *Evaluating Early Intervention Programs for Severely Handicapped Children and Their Families*, Pro-ed, Austin.

Bricker, D. D. (1986) *Early Education of At-risk Handicapped Infants, Toddlers, and Preschool Children*, Scott, Foresman, Glenview.

Bromwich, R. M. (1981) *Working with Parents*, University Park Press, Baltimore.

Brynelsen, D. (ed.) (1984) *Working Together: A Handbook for Parents and Professionals*, British Columbians for Mentally Handicapped People, Vancouver.

Dokecki, P. R. (1986) 'The Impact of Evaluation Research on Policy Making,' in L. Bickman and D. L. Weatherford (eds), *Evaluating Early Intervention Programs for Severely Handicapped Children and Their Families*, Pro-ed, Austin.

Dunst, C.J. (1985) 'Overview of the Efficacy of Early Intervention Programs: Methodological and Conceptual Considerations' in L. Bickman and D.L. Weatherford (eds), *Evaluating Early Intervention Programs for Severely Handicapped Children and Their Families*, Pro-ed, Austin.

Fewell, R. R. (1983) 'The Team Approach to Infant Education,' in S. G. Garwood and R. R. Fewell (eds), *Educating Handicapped Infants: Issues in Development and Intervention*, Aspen, Rockville, Maryland.

Fewell, R. R. (1986) 'The Measurement of Family Functioning,' in L. Bickman and D. L. Weatherford (eds), *Evaluating Early Intervention Programs for Severely Handicapped Children and Their Families*, Pro-ed, Austin.

Filler, J. W. (1983) 'Service Models for Handicapped Infants,' in S. G. Garwood and R. R. Fewell (eds), *Educating Handicapped Infants: Issues in Development and Intervention*, Aspen, Rockville, Maryland.

Gabel, H., McDowell, J., and Cerreto, M. C. (1983) 'Family Adaptation to the Handicapped Infant,' in S. G. Garwood and R. R. Fewell (eds), *Educating Handicapped Infants: Issues in Development and Intervention*, Aspen, Rockville, Maryland.

Guralnick, M. J. and Bennett, F. C. (eds) (1987) *The Effectiveness of Early Intervention for At-risk and Handicapped Children*, Academic Press, Orlando.

Guralnick, M. J. and Bricker, D. (1987) 'The Effectiveness of Early Intervention for Children with Cognitive and General Developmental Delays,' in M. J. Guralnick & F. C. Bennett (eds), *The Effec-*

tiveness of Early Intervention for At-risk and Handicapped Children, Academic Press, Orlando.

Honig, A. S. (1982) 'Infant–mother Communication', *Young Children*, 37, 52–62.

Hosaka, C. M. (1984) 'Summary Report on the Status of Curriculum Development for the Kupulani Project,' *Early Education Bulletin*, *No. 17*, Center for Development of Early Education, Kamehameha Schools/Bernice Pauahi Bishop Estate, Honolulu.

Hughson, E.A. and Brown, R.I. (1988) ' Evaluation of Adult Rehabilitation Programmes,' *Irish Journal of Psychology*, 9, 249–263.

Hupp, S. C. and Kaiser, A. P. (1986) 'Evaluating Educational Programs for Severely Handicapped Preschoolers,' in L. Bickman and D. L. Weatherford (eds), *Evaluating Early Intervention Programs for Severely Handicapped Children and Their Families*, Pro-ed, Austin.

Kemmis, S. and McTaggart, R. (1982) *The Action Research Planner*, Deakin University Press, Deakin.

Kysela, G. M., McDonald, L., Reddon, J. and Gobeil-Dwyer, F. (1987) 'Stress and Supports to Families with a Handicapped Child,' in K. Marfo (ed.), *Mental Handicap and Parent-Child Interactions*, Praeger, New York.

Lillie, D. (1981) 'Educational and Psychological Strategies for Working with Parents,' in J. L. Paul (ed.), *Understanding and Working with Parents of Children with Special Needs*, Holt, Rinehart and Winston, New York.

Mannino, F. V. and Shore, M. F. (1985) 'Understanding Consultation: Some Orientating Dimensions,' *The Counseling Psychologist*, 13.

Manolson, A. (1983) *It Takes Two to Talk: A Hanen Early Language Parent Guide Book*, Hanen Early Language Resource Centre, Toronto.

Marfo, K. and Kysela, G. M. (1985) 'Early Intervention with Mentally Handicapped Children: A Critical Appraisal of Applied Research,' *Journal of Pediatric Psychology*, 10, 305–324.

Mitchell, D. R. (1983) 'International Trends in Special Education,' *Canadian Journal of Mental Retardation*, 33, 6–13.

Mitchell, D. R. (1986) 'A Developmental Systems Approach to Planning and Evaluating Services for Persons with Handicaps,' in R.I. Brown (ed.), *Management and Administration of Rehabilitation Programmes*, Croom Helm, London.

Mitchell, D. R. (1987) 'Parents' Interactions with Their Developmentally Disabled or At-risk Infants: A Focus for Intervention,' *Australia and New Zealand Journal of Developmental Disabilities*, 12.

Mitchell, D., Brynelsen, D., and Holm, M. (1988) 'Evaluating the Process of Early Intervention Programmes,' *Irish Journal of Psychology*, 9.

Mittler, P., Mittler, H. and McConachie, H. (1986) *Working Together: Guidelines for Partnership between Professionals and Parents of Children and Young People with Disabilities*, UNESCO, Paris.

Orelove, F. and Sobsey, D. (1987) *Educating Children with Multiple Disabilities: A Transdisciplinary Approach*, Brookes, Baltimore.

Peterson, N. L. (1987) *Early Intervention for Handicapped and At-risk Children*, Love, Denver.

Pieterse, M. (1985) 'The Macquarie Program for Developmentally Delayed Preschool Children: Minimum Requirements for Evaluating the Program', *Working Paper*, School of Education, Macquarie University, Sydney.

Rosenberg, S. A. and Robinson, C. C. (1985) 'Enhancement of Mothers' Interactional Skills in an Infant Education Program,' *Education and Training of the Mentally Retarded, 20,* 163–169.

Seligman, M. (ed.) (1983) *The Family with a Handicapped Child: Understanding and Treatment*, Grune and Stratton, New York.

Shadish, W. R. (1986) 'Sources of Evaluation Practice: Needs, Purposes, Questions and Technology,'in L. Bickman and D. L. Weatherford (eds), *Evaluating Early Intervention Programs for Severely Handicapped Children and Their Families*, Pro-ed, Austin.

Smith, N.L. (1986) 'Evaluation Alternatives for Early Intervention Programs,'in L. Bickman and D. L. Weatherford (eds), *Evaluating Early Intervention Programs for Severely Handicapped Children and Their Families*, Pro-ed, Austin

Straton, E. A. (1985) 'Early Intervention Services,' in N. N. Singh and K. M. Wilton (eds), *Mental Retardation in New Zealand: Provisions, Services and Research*, Whitcoulls, Christchurch, New Zealand.

Sub-regional Workshop for Commonwealth Countries of South-East-Central Africa (1987) *Recommendations Adopted on Early Intervention to Prevent or Ameliorate Mental Handicap and Developmental Disabilities*, University of Zambia, Lusaka.

US Department of Education (1987) 'Early Intervention Program for Infants and Toddlers with Handicaps; Notice of Proposed Rulemaking,' *Federal Register, 52,* No. 222, November, Washington, DC.

Vincent, L., Tooke, A., Fredericks, B., Baldwin, V., Zeitlin, S., Smith, B., Black, T., and Woodruff, G. (1986) 'Testimony Supports Early Intervention (Statement to US House of Representatives' Sub-Committee on Select Education, on Behalf of TASH, the CEDH Division for Early Childhood and Interact — The National Committee for Young Children with Special Needs and Their Families), *TASH Newsletter*.

Warnock, M. (Chair) (1978) *Special Education Needs: Report of Committee of Inquiry into the Education of Handicapped Children*, HMSO, London.

Westby, C. E. (1988) 'Cultural Differences in Caregiver — Child Interaction: Implications for Assessment and Intervention,' in L. Cole and V. Deal (eds), *Communication Disorders in Multicultural Populations*, ASHA, Rockville.

Wolery, M. and Bailey, D. B. (1984) 'Alternatives to Impact Evaluations: Suggestions for Program Evaluation in Early Intervention,' *Journal of the Division for Early Childhood, 9*, 26–37.

Author Index